"After thirty-plus years of 'diets' and in the midst of the most dire overweigl history, including a record number of message is clear: diets don't work! What is important is an intelligent way of eating, which is a lifestyle predominated by living food that allows the eating experience to remain a joyous one, not a clinical endeavor. *Never Be Fat Again* succeeds in giving the reader a simple, straightforward, commonsense approach to eating that fulfills that lofty goal."

—Harvey Diamond
Author, *Fit for Life*

"This is not just another 'dime a dozen' diet book. *Never Be Fat Again* hits the nail on the head. This book provides scientifically authenticated information combined with the practical help necessary to answer the problem of overweight that is rampant in our society. As director at Hippocrates Health Institute for thirty-plus years, I can attest to the fact that a plant-based, living-foods diet, without toxic processed food, when combined with other lifestyle changes, brings dramatic and lasting results. Lifestyle is the name of the game, and I believe that employing the wealth of information represented in this book will help you change your life for the better."

—Brian Clement, N.M.D., Ph.D.
Director, Hippocrates Health Institute

"*Never Be Fat Again* goes far beyond traditional mainstream tactics that blame the patient for being overweight. Raymond Francis translates complex cutting-edge biochemistry into easy-to-read, practical strategies that will help anyone win the battle of the bulge. Unlike the hundreds of low-calorie diets that don't work, Francis addresses the underlying causes of what slows our metabolism and drives us to overeat. This book is a must-read for anyone who wants to lose weight and keep it off, as well as for those people who have tried and failed dozens of times."

—Len Saputo, M.D.
Medical Director, Health Medicine Institute

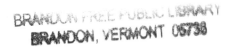

"It's not how much you eat, but the hidden toxins in your diet that may be making you gain weight. Learn how to not only lose weight but gain back your health! Full of practical and scientifically based information, this book is a user-friendly guide to a healthy lifestyle and permanent weight loss."

—**Hyla Cass, M.D.**
Author, *8 Weeks to Vibrant Health*

"Americans are facing serious dangers never before experienced in history. Our population is eating itself to death with a toxic diet, and Raymond Francis steps up to the dinner plate and hits a home run."

—**Joel Fuhrman, M.D.**
Bestselling author, *Disease-Proof Your Child* and *Eat to Live*

"This book is your indispensable stepping stone to unchanging Truth about human nutritional needs. History tells us that only Truth will never change. Over many years I have watched diets come and go. There is but one diet for humans, not only for weight loss, but for ideal health. I call it the Living Foods Diet and have written extensively about it in *Second Opinion*. Does it work? I haven't yet seen one overweight person who follows this diet. Read *Never Be Fat Again,* follow it, and you can reclaim control over your weight and health from the disease-producing factories and industries that thrive on your sicknesses."

—**Robert Jay Rowen, M.D.**
Editor in Chief, *Second Opinion*
www.secondopinionnewsletter.com

"*Never Be Fat Again* is a light of hope to many who struggle with the disease of overweight and obesity. Raymond Francis's vision of a trim, disease-free, healthy America needs to become everyone's vision at a time when chronic disease is epidemic. I salute his inner spirit, which is guiding millions worldwide. If you want to unfold the ultimate truth about your weight issue and be a visionary of your perfect self, read this book."

—**Su Jain, M.D.**
Medical Director, Mt. Diablo Wellness Center

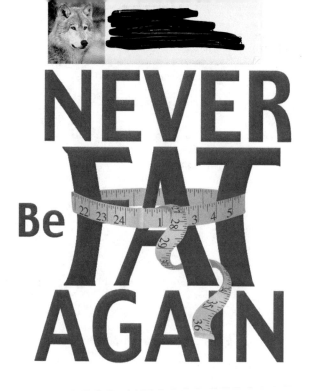

NEVER
Be FAT
AGAIN

The **6-WEEK** Cellular **SOLUTION** to Permanently Break the Fat Cycle

RAYMOND FRANCIS, D.Sc.
Author of Never Be Sick Again
and Michelle King

Health Communications, Inc.
Deerfield Beach, Florida

www.hcibooks.com

Never Be Fat Again and the information contained in this book are not intended as a substitute for the advice and/or medical care of the reader's physician, nor are they meant to discourage or dissuade the reader from the advice of his or her physician. The reader should regularly consult with a physician in matters relating to his or her health, and especially with regard to symptoms that may require diagnosis. Any eating or lifestyle regimen should be undertaken under the direct supervision of the reader's physician. Moreover, anyone with chronic or serious ailments should undertake any eating and lifestyle program, and/or changes to his or her personal eating and lifestyle regimen, under the direct supervision of his or her physician. If the reader has any questions concerning the information presented in this book, or its application to his or her particular medical profile, or if the reader has unusual medical or nutritional needs or constraints that may conflict with the advice in this book, he or she should consult his or her physician. If the reader is pregnant or nursing she should consult her physician before embarking on any nutrition or lifestyle program.

Library of Congress Cataloging-in-Publication Data

Francis, Raymond.
Never be fat again : the 6-week cellular solution to permanently break the fat cycle / Raymond Francis and Michelle King.
p. cm.
Includes bibliographical references and index.
ISBN-13: ISBN 978-0-7573-0531-3 (trade paper)
ISBN-10: ISBN 0-7573-0531-8 (trade paper)
1. Nutrition. 2. Diet. 3. Health. 4. Weight loss—Psychological aspects.
I. King, Michelle. II. Title.
RA784.F66 2007
613.2—dc22

2006033442

Publisher: Health Communications, Inc.
3201 S.W. 15th Street
Deerfield Beach, FL 33442-8190

Cover design by Larissa Hise Henoch
Inside design and formatting by Dawn Von Strolley Grove

Contents

Acknowledgments

I would like to acknowledge with grateful appreciation all of those who have helped to make this book a reality. To accomplish a project such as this, one must be shaped, inspired, influenced, motivated, supported, and schooled by a great many people, who I now acknowledge and thank. Quality work requires quality people, and I have been blessed with many in the creation of this book. First and foremost, I would like to thank my wonderful publisher, Health Communications, Inc. HCI is a national treasure for all the wonderful information it has made available to the public. Most especially, I would like to express my heartfelt thanks to its vice president and general manager, Tom Sand. Tom's support, inspiration, sage advice, and friendship were instrumental in making this book possible. I would also like to thank my HCI editors, Allison Janse and Bob Land, along with all the other wonderful people at HCI who helped in the production and marketing of this book.

I also wish to acknowledge and thank my other editors: Linda Hall, Pamela Strong, and Joan Carole, whose critiques and insightful comments helped to make this work more readable. My thanks would not be complete without acknowledging and expressing my gratitude to the many people who read and commented on drafts of this manuscript as it evolved.

These include Dr. Russell Blaylock, Bernard Friesecke, Pascal Girard, Brianna Grigsby, Dr. Linda Howard, Philip Jacklin, Dr. Russell Jaffe, Austin and Georgene King, Diane Lahoski, JoAnne Williams, Robert Menkemeller, Mollie Meyers, Jamie Romeo, Dr. David Rovno, Brandon Soule, and Nancy Talbot.

I wish to particularly acknowledge my coauthor, Michelle King. Many thanks, Michelle, for the inspiration, countless nights and weekends, and dedication that helped to make this book a reality—and special thanks for the wonderful recipe chapter.

—Raymond Francis

Foreword

The obesity crisis can never be solved without correctly defining the problem. *Never Be Fat Again* defines the problem correctly for the first time: overweight is a disease that can be cured only by restoring overall good health. It then proceeds to offer a comprehensive lifestyle solution for restoring health, not only nutritionally but toxicologically, psychologically, physically, genetically, and medically.

This is one of the most important books you can read on the subject of health and weight control. Not only will it help you achieve your ideal weight, but more than that, it will help you live a long and healthy life, free from the chronic diseases that are epidemic in our society.

Throughout my many years of medical practice and studying nutritional science, I had never read a "diet" book that I thought was worth reading—much less following—until *Never Be Fat Again*. Most of these books, written by self-promoters and hucksters, lack any credible scientific foundation. A few include some valid scientific principles, but they never address the total health picture. Weight loss, by any means possible, is the obsession.

What makes *Never Be Fat Again* different and better is that Raymond Francis and Michelle King put the horse before the cart. They direct our attention first and foremost to something far more important than weight loss: regaining and maintaining health! But not to worry. As health is regained, the loss of unwanted pounds follows *as a natural consequence.*

What does this mean about the quality of your life? Instead of feeling deprived and exhausted as you lose excess pounds, you feel satisfied and invigorated! Wouldn't you rather do it the easy and enjoyable way? In my own experience with helping others achieve optimal health, I've seen this weight loss "side effect" time and time again, and I can tell you without any doubt that putting health first not only works, it is the only intelligent way to lose weight.

People have been misled by a massive campaign of propaganda to see fat loss as being synonymous with good health, no matter how it is done. In this book you will learn, maybe for the first time, why such a policy is a sure road to disaster. Everyone knows that most diet plans don't work long term because they aren't sustainable. Few realize how unhealthy these diets can be. Yo-yo dieting is extremely dangerous and can lead to a number of serious chronic diseases. Very-low-calorie dieting can cause smoldering, unrecognized diseases to surface; you may lose weight, but you experience failing health. Severe caloric restriction as well as extremely high protein or fat intake can lead to muscle damage—not only in the limbs, but in vital organs such as the heart, liver, and kidneys. Heart and kidney failure are both major hazards of strenuous dieting. These kinds of diet plans have disappointed millions, and they won't work for you.

The publication of *Never Be Fat Again* couldn't be more timely. Americans are floundering in our attempts to deal with our obesity crisis. During the period 1976–1980, it was estimated that 47.4 percent of Americans were overweight or obese. Today, some 65.2 percent of adults and over 40 percent of children are in this category. People have become so desperate to lose weight that in 2001 some 47,000 major surgeries were done to reverse obesity. Last year that figure jumped to

145,000. Shockingly, 1,400 of these people died on the operating table. And thousands of others in search of weight loss wound up with heart damage from the weight-loss drug Fen-Phen.

Raymond Francis is one of the few scientists to achieve a breakthrough understanding of health and disease. His theory that there is really only one disease with two causes—deficiency of needed nutrients and toxicity—is as profound as it is simple. To build health (and lose weight) he tells us to eat *more*—more nutrients, that is. There is tremendous power in getting rid of the "fake foods" and eating real, nutritious food. And he makes an even more unique and essential contribution in his attention to toxins.

Do toxins make you fat? You bet they do! And toxins are everywhere in the Standard American Diet. "Bad fats," pesticides, herbicides, toxic metals, MSG, aspartame, and a long list of other harmful processed food ingredients, hormones, antibiotics, and bacterial and viral contaminants all pollute our foods. Extensive research shows that some toxins, even in very minute concentrations (millionths of a gram), can severely disrupt cell function, leading to sickness, including obesity, and even death. Shockingly, a large number of legally permitted food additives have never been adequately tested for safety, and almost none have been tested together to see what happens when they are combined. You need the information on toxins in this book—not only to lose weight but to survive living in the twenty-first century! The information on toxins alone is worth the price.

I am impressed with the broad scope of this unique book. The authors explain to the reader why each change in diet is critical to regaining health and achieving desired fat loss. I think omitting this information is a flaw of so many books. If you have no clear understanding as to why you should avoid certain foods, eat certain portions, and include other foods in your diet, you are unlikely to follow through over the long term.

I was also pleased to see that the authors discuss the role of excess fat in the development of chronic diseases. Weight loss is no longer just a cosmetic consideration. There is compelling evidence that obesity, especially fat around the middle, plays a critical role in a number of diseases, such as type 2 diabetes; heart disease; autoimmune diseases; neurological diseases like Alzheimer's, Parkinson's, and ALS; and metabolic syndrome (a newly defined condition that combines obesity with heart disease *and* diabetes).

There is growing evidence that virtually every disease is made worse by excessive body fat, especially abdominal fat. We now know that special fat cells secrete powerful inflammatory chemicals that damage cells, organs, and tissues all over the body, including the brain, heart, liver, eyes, and kidneys. Yet, as the authors point out, if you lose the fat the wrong way you can make things worse because you further weaken your cells and prevent their recovery.

Losing excess fat is essential, not just for adults, but also for our children. Yet we must resist quick-fix diets and gimmicks that lead only to losing health and ultimately regaining lost fat. What is needed is a lifestyle plan that gives you the knowledge necessary to lose weight, gain health, and look and feel great for the rest of your life. *Never Be Fat Again* provides such a comprehensive healthcare system that is based on scientifically sound principles for creating and maintaining lifelong health, including a healthy weight. It is not an exaggeration to say that *Never Be Fat Again* can transform your body and your life in a miraculous way simply by supplying you with the truth you've been starving for!

Russell L. Blaylock, M.D.

Dr. Blaylock is a retired neurosurgeon and presently a professor of biology. He is the author of *Excitotoxins: The Taste That Kills; Health and Nutrition Secrets That Can Save Your Life; Natural Strategies for Cancer Patients;* and *The Blaylock Wellness Report.*

Introduction

Most overweight people feel helpless. They have tried everything; they have lost the same pounds again and again. Many have given up hope. But there is hope! Permanent weight loss is possible—if you know how to do it. The key is to understand that overweight is a disease, caused by malnutrition and environmental toxins. Weight-loss diets don't work because you cannot cure this disease by trying to lose weight. The weight is merely a symptom, and this symptom will come back unless you eliminate the underlying causes.

Chances are you want to lose weight. If you want to lose weight, do not go on a diet, at least not a diet as we have come to know that word—deprivation, aggravation, even starvation. To lose weight *permanently*, not just while you are suffering through another silly, trendy, latest/greatest "diet," you must understand that overweight is a disease, not a cosmetic flaw. Once you learn the true causes of this disease, you can heal yourself and regain health, energy, and a more youthful appearance.

Never Be Fat Again is fundamentally different from your typical weight-loss book. It is not about an on-again, off-again diet. In fact, it is not about a diet at all. It is about a way of living that works with your body and not against it. In truth, there is no such thing as a popular "diet" that works in the long term. Such diets trick the body into quick but temporary weight loss by putting it in an unnatural and unhealthy state. This book gives you the keys to good health and permanent weight loss by showing you how to live a lifestyle that is based on the most recent advances in science as well as on thousands of years of biological history. Unlike the iffy science in your usual weight-loss book, the long-term effectiveness of this weight-controlling, health-giving lifestyle is a proven fact. We know it works!

In this book, we tell you how low-fat and no-fat products can actually make you fatter. We show you how a missing nutrient can signal your body to store fat. We also expose the truth about how common chemical toxins, found in most foods, alter the expression of weight-control genes and can pack on pounds. Your body already knows how to balance its weight. You just have to give your body a fighting chance.

Just about everyone dreams of staying trim and looking younger. Billions of dollars are spent every year on diet plans, books, gimmicks, and tricks, but without an understanding of how your body chemistry works, you are sabotaging your own efforts. In fact, you might actually be causing yourself to gain more weight as well as to damage your health. Losing weight is a national obsession, yet the public continues to lack clearly defined scientific guidelines to deal with this problem. Obesity rates are skyrocketing. Americans rank among the sickest people in the industrialized world, and life expectancy is about to turn down. Weight-loss diets and programs have failed us because they are scientifically and nutritionally unsound.

The cutting-edge science in this book remains unknown to most people because new scientific knowledge often takes a half-century or more to reach the general public. Even modern medicine has yet to translate these discoveries into clinical practice. Not surprisingly, powerful commercial interests don't want you to know the truth about the American diet and the magnitude of the disaster it has created. These interests are actively working to suppress this information by obscuring it in a fog of misleading junk science and food-industry propaganda.

Eat Plenty and Lose Weight

Perhaps in the past you managed to lose weight by going on a popular diet plan, but you did not, in fact, cure your overweight disease. Your weight was destined to return. You cannot lose weight permanently by trying to lose weight. To be successful, you must restore your health first; that is the engine that will drive weight loss, including dramatic weight loss. You don't have to work at losing weight because it will happen automatically if you address the underlying causes. All you have to do is provide yourself with good nutrition and avoid toxins. Sounds too simple? In so many ways it is simple. Don't get us wrong: you may have to make significant changes in your lifestyle, but you do not need to suffer. And your rewards can be exhilarating.

Erase your old definition of "diet"—the negative one. Think of your new lifestyle in a positive, appealing, even exciting new way. Consuming the total nutrition your body needs to stay well is automatically a plan for losing and keeping off excess weight. Feed your body the right foods (and plenty of them) and keep away from the toxic and nutritionally deficient foodstuffs sitting on supermarket shelves, and your body will regulate itself.

Healthy weight isn't just about looking good; it is about

living well—fewer illnesses (ideally, no illness at all), clearer arteries, fewer disabilities, and a longer life. Excess body weight is a risk factor for health problems that include cancer, diabetes, hypertension, heart disease, and more, not to mention fatigue and accelerated aging. When you have excess weight you move slower, you tire faster, you feel worse. Indeed, a healthy body is also a more beautiful body: glowing skin, fewer wrinkles, better hair. In fact, you can reverse aging effects that have already occurred; you can reverse diseases from which you already suffer.

From Disaster to Wisdom: Raymond's Story

I have counseled overweight and chronically ill patients for two decades, and I have seen people who had failed at countless diets lose weight and regain their health. I have seen some amazing transformations with even cancer patients and other terminally ill individuals getting a new lease on life. All of these people had something in common. With my help, they came to understand what really causes disease, and they realized there is a solution to almost any disease.

I had to realize this on my own when I was forced to save my life from certain death. At the age of forty-eight, I was president of an international management consulting firm when my life was devastated by illness, including three autoimmune syndromes, chronic fatigue, and chemical sensitivity syndromes. Through a series of epic blunders by the physicians who treated me, I nearly died of liver failure. After causing my health crisis, these physicians announced that there was nothing more they could do. Essentially, I was left for dead, dying of chemical hepatitis caused by a prescription drug. At six foot two, I had been reduced to a skeletal 120 pounds. In this state of weakness, unable to even lift my head from the pillow, I searched for answers. I relied on my training as a chemist and my knowledge of biochemistry, and began a journey toward health. I began by taking megadoses of vitamin C. Within twenty-four hours of supplementing with vitamin C, my vital signs began to stabilize. By the second day I could sit up in bed. Amazed by the power of even one nutrient to heal, I thus began a long road to recovery and a life newly dedicated to studying what makes people sick and how to make them healthy again.

I am now seventy years old and have been told by my physicians that I have the health of a much younger man. I never get colds or flu. I am the same weight I was at twenty. I get frequent compliments on how good my skin looks. Recently my arteries were measured, and I have the arteries of a thirty-year-old. The biological age of my arteries is less than half my chronological age, and my risk of having a stroke or heart attack is that of a thirty-year-old. Why are my arteries so healthy? I made the necessary changes in diet and lifestyle that allowed my arteries to repair and reverse aging and disease. You can learn how to do this too. You can learn how to reduce your biological age and literally become younger. As you become younger and healthier, you will also achieve normal weight. Over the last two decades, as I have worked with clients to help them overcome their health problems, I noticed that weight loss occurred as a side effect of good health. Further, the weight loss was permanent. Since I now know that overweight is a disease, it is not a surprise that good health equals normal weight.

It took two years to restore my health. During that time, I came to realize that conventional medicine focused on disease. Medicine has no understanding of health and little to offer the sick; instead of curing disease, all it does is manage disease by treating the symptoms. I didn't want my diseases managed; I wanted them cured. I came to realize that health was a choice, but that someone without my scientific knowledge would probably have a difficult time making this choice. It also became clear that most of the supplements and health products on the market were of low quality and some even dangerous. It was then that I decided to devote the remainder of my life to researching health and teaching others how to get well and stay well.

In 1994, I started a company called Beyond Health. The purpose of Beyond Health is to help people go "beyond health" as they have known it, so they can get well, stay well, and never be sick again. Beyond Health does this by supplying the public with an advanced healthcare system consisting of a unique health model, cutting-edge health information, and carefully researched, world-class, safe, and effective health-supporting products. In that same year, I also started the Beyond Health radio show (which can be heard worldwide, 24/7 at www.beyondhealth.com by clicking on "Radio") and a newsletter, *Beyond Health News*. I lecture all over the world, and in September 2002, my first book, *Never Be Sick Again,* was published. In 2003, it was nominated for "best health book" and the prestigious Nautilus Award by the publishing industry. In it, I outlined a new model of health—the Beyond Health Model based on the concept of one disease, two causes, and six pathways. This is a revolutionary new way of thinking about health and disease that focuses on eliminating the true causes of disease. The model is so simple that almost anyone can understand it, and yet so powerful that people around the world have been able to heal themselves of incurable diseases after learning it.

The newest manifestation of my health odyssey is the *Never Be Fat Again* Lifestyle (*NBFA* Lifestyle), a new approach to weight control—fighting fat as a disease. This new approach recognizes only one disease—that is, malfunctioning cells (cells are the individual building blocks out of which our bodies are made). This disease has two causes—a deficiency of what cells need to function normally and toxicity resulting from exposure to substances that disrupt normal cell function. Very simply, overweight is a disease that stems from malfunctioning cells, caused by deficiency and toxicity, resulting in excess weight.

If every cell in your body is functioning normally, you cannot be sick or overweight. Like any other disease, overweight can be prevented and reversed. Viewing all sicknesses as one disease with two causes removes the mystery and puts the power over disease into the hands of the individual. Indeed, cellular medicine—maintaining and restoring cellular health—will become the medical model of the twenty-first century. It will replace the obsolete, ineffective, and unscientific system of medicine in current use, wherein medical specialists diagnose a myriad of different diseases and treat the symptoms instead of the causes. As a scientist who sees the implications of these wonderful new discoveries regarding cellular health, my goal is to provide you with the knowledge you need to understand your predicament and a road map for getting to where you want to go—toward good health and normal weight.

To help you implement this lifestyle, this book offers Six Pathways that you can employ as weapons in fighting fat as a disease with the goal of improving your health. As your cells undergo transformation, your health will also undergo transformation. You will begin to lose weight and produce more energy.

We encourage you to read the chapters of *Never Be Fat Again* in the order they appear, and to resist the temptation to skip over theory and go right to the eating plan and recipes. Reading this book will empower you to change your thinking and be liberated from dieting to a lifestyle focused on living and eating for health. This is a life-changing journey. Follow this strategy and you will feel different and look different, you will live better and longer, and you will have health, energy, and vitality. You will be a new you. You will never want to go back to your old ways.

PART I

The Foundation for Living the *NBFA* Lifestyle

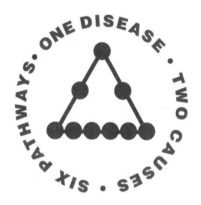

Fundamental to living the health-giving, body-slimming lifestyle described in this book is an understanding of why it works. In order to grasp this, you have to realize that overweight is actually a disease, not just a cosmetic problem, and it has two primary causes—deficiency and toxicity. A disease can only be conquered by addressing its root causes. Most weight-loss plans use futile Band-Aid approaches designed to produce rapid weight loss without addressing the underlying causes of overweight. Part I helps you to identify the real causes so you can stop merely attacking the symptom of excess pounds. As a disease, overweight can be defeated using the six weapons, called the Six Pathways, which are briefly introduced here and then explained in greater detail in the remainder of the book.

FIGHTING FAT AS A DISEASE

In any battle it is critical to understand the enemy in order to win. This chapter gives you breakthrough information about fat and how to control it. Such knowledge is the essential foundation for winning your personal battle against overweight. Among the information you'll learn in this chapter:

- Overweight is a disease that disrupts your body chemistry, causing other disorders.
- The problem in fighting this battle is not usually a lack of willpower, but the lack of a clear understanding about how cellular malfunction causes overweight.
- There are two main causes of this malfunction:
  1. Lack of nutrients (yes, you can be overweight while your cells are starving for nutrition)
  2. Toxins (yes, we inadvertently poison ourselves daily, which can make us fat)

• There are six major weapons we need to fight fat—nutrition, toxic avoidance, healthy thought patterns, physical maintenance, awareness of how we can control our genes, and discernment when choosing or refusing medical options.

What is especially exciting about nutrition is not just the possibility of prevention, but the reversal of diseases. The body has a tremendous ability to heal itself. . . .

—Russell L. Blaylock
Health and Nutrition Secrets

After nearly a lifetime of being overweight, Melissa, age forty-eight, looked fat, old, and tired. She was clinically obese and chronically depressed, and on some days she even wanted to end her life. Although she had read dozens of weight-loss books and tried even more "diets," she remained prediabetic and chronically fatigued, and she suffered skin problems and hair loss. She reached a crossroads. She chose a new path, and she changed her life. That new path is the guide to wellness and weight loss offered in this book. After eighteen months of living the lifestyle you will learn about—the *Never Be Fat Again* Lifestyle—Melissa looked substantially younger, her figure was slim and toned, her skin radiant, and her hair healthy—a complete turnaround. "I am an entirely different person," she said "and nobody is more surprised than my family. I think I have reversed the clock by fifteen years, and I have lost so much weight people don't recognize me. My depression and fatigue are gone, an old surgery scar has disappeared, and I have energy to spare."

Melissa's struggles were not unique, and her remarkable

transformation need not be extraordinary either. This kind of weight loss and reversal of overweight disease is within your reach. The catalyst for change in Melissa's life was her realization that all her health problems, including her overweight, actually had the same two causes: deficiency and toxicity. Her body was getting too few of the right things and too many of the wrong things. Despite her sacrifices, Melissa's "diets" had been sabotaging her health and standing in the way of successful weight loss.

To lose weight, you do not need a host of medical specialists, "diet" gimmicks, or "diet" foods. *Losing weight is not about how to lose weight; it is about how to regain health.* You can achieve normal weight without counting calories, without feeling hungry or deprived, and without going on an unnatural "diet" that will actually harm your health. In order to accomplish this, however, you need to understand how your body works and why it sometimes becomes diseased.

You Cannot Be Healthy and Overweight

New research indicates that overweight is a chronic disease that disrupts normal body chemistry, accelerates aging, and causes a wide variety of disabilities and health problems, including cancer. Numerous studies have proven that overweight people suffer from higher rates of cancer, heart disease, high blood pressure, diabetes, high cholesterol and triglycerides, breathing disorders, sleep disorders, arthritis, asthma, kidney stones, premature aging, and early death. Obese mothers are more than twice as likely to have children with debilitating birth defects. If you are overweight, your life expectancy is reduced.

Very simply, lean people live longer and have less disease, less disability, more energy, and a higher quality of life. Cosmetic considerations aside, this is why maintaining normal weight is so very important. A number of studies, including the Nurses Health Study, a large ongoing health study that began in 1976, have shown that the leanest 20 percent live the longest, with mortality increasing progressively for each added pound. Perhaps even more important than living longer, lean people have higher-quality lives because they suffer less disability and dependence on others. Even if you have gained only ten pounds since high school, you are at risk for increased health problems, more disability, and shorter life.

Healthy people are not overweight, and overweight people are never truly healthy. In fact, new studies indicate that predicting long-term health may be as simple as taking a waist measurement. Fat around the waist has been linked to higher mortality and the long list of diseases cited above. But the good news is that even modest weight loss can have significant health benefits, among which are improved balance of triglycerides, cholesterol, and blood sugar. Some diabetics even go off insulin. Your body has an amazing ability to self-regulate, self-repair, and heal; you just have to give it a fighting chance.

Your body is programmed to regulate appetite, fat storage, fat burning, and weight, along with body temperature, blood pressure, blood sugar, hormone balance, and thousands of other functions. *Your* job is to help your body to do its job. When you interfere with the body's self-regulating systems by making yourself deficient and toxic, you *will* get sick—guaranteed.

Deficiency and toxicity, the two causes of disease, affect weight by interfering with your appetite and weight-control functions. Exercise also has a huge effect on these control mechanisms and is essential. Maintaining normal appetite and fat-storing controls are critical to controlling your weight. These controls are not just about willpower; they are about biology. They depend on the normal functioning of your cells, and when these mechanisms are disturbed, you can gain weight, no matter what you eat. Think what would happen if your appetite and fat-storage controls were stuck in the "on" position: you would eat a lot and get fat. Even if you eat fewer calories, you can still get fat if your cells are being instructed to store fat.

Nutrient deficiency stimulates appetite, causes hunger and cravings, and signals the body to store fat. Toxins can have the same effect as nutrient deficiency; they cause appetite to stay in the "on" position, as well as signal the body to store fat. No matter how hard you try, long-term normal weight cannot be achieved without eliminating deficiency and toxicity. Failure to address these issues is why popular diets work only in the short term; they fail to correct the true causes of overweight.

When we gain weight, our first thought is that we should eat less. The truth is we should eat more, because we are actually suffering from malnutrition. The catch is we have to eat more of the right foods, foods that are rich in essential nutrients. Most people, though, are confused about what is good for them and what is not. One day we are told to switch from butter to margarine; then we are told that margarine is bad for us. On another day, we are told to switch to high-carb diets, and on another to low-carb diets. We are told to switch from saturated to polyunsaturated fats only to find later that the polyunsaturated fats are causing an epidemic of cancer, heart disease, and obesity. We are told that coffee and chocolate are bad, and then we are told they are good. We are told that vitamin E is good for the heart, and then we are told falsely that it is not. No wonder people end up sticking to their familiar diet and lifestyle. Many go on to try one fad diet after another, all of which include make-believe foods guaranteed to make you sick.

Lack of Willpower Isn't the Problem

Overweight is often viewed as evidence of inadequacy, weakness, and lack of willpower—that is, as a character flaw.

We think that overweight people eat too much and don't exercise enough; all they have to do to be slim is eat less and exercise more. But this is not true. Even if you have enough willpower to keep yourself from eating, you still may not lose weight.

Most clients who have come to us for nutritional advice regarding their weight problems are highly motivated. Often they have tried numerous diets and gimmicks, but they failed. More than 95 percent of those who try traditional "diet" plans regain any lost weight within the first two years, and many gain back more than they lost.

Warning: The Standard American Diet Is a Hazard

The Standard American Diet is our leading cause of disease—a diet of chronic disease and death. *It is virtually impossible to consume such a diet and be healthy or trim.* So stop trying to do the impossible and then expecting that a magic shake, a pill that melts fat away while you sleep, or your doctor will solve your problems.

The Standard American Diet is loaded with more calories than we can use. Whenever we consume more calories than necessary to maintain our current weight, we store fat. Our biology is designed for the life of the hunter-gatherer. Historically, hunter-gathers might go for days without food. When they found food, they would gorge themselves because they didn't know where their next meal was coming from. The excess calories were stored as fat to supply them with energy when food was scarce.

Throughout human history, our biggest concern was to obtain enough food. Now we live a lifestyle with an abundance of inexpensive, calorie-rich, nutritionally inadequate food that is vastly different from the diet to which our bodies are biologically adapted. The Standard American Diet contains health-damaging sugar, salt, white flour, and dairy, too much animal protein, and the wrong fats, providing insufficient nutrients and excessive toxins. Meanwhile, technology has made our lives easier, so we engage in less physical activity than ever, expending little energy. There are ever-present ads for timesaving convenience foods (i.e., junk foods). The pace of life seems to go faster and faster, leaving less time to prepare the wholesome foods that people were eating just decades ago. This diet and lifestyle send inappropriate instructions to our genes, stimulate our bodies to store excess calories as fat, accelerate aging, and result in malnutrition. Eating mostly high-calorie junk food while not doing a lot of physical work is a surefire formula for gaining weight.

Our biological ancestors were *not* overweight. They did not have an endless supply of food available, and the amount of nutrition and fiber in the natural foods they were eating was sufficient to fill their stomachs, satisfy their nutritional needs, and shut off their appetite. They also were not exposed to man-made toxins that interfered with their appetite and fat-storing controls. Moreover, they engaged in a lot of physically demanding activity. The body has an exquisite system for balancing caloric intake with energy expenditure, shutting off the appetite when we have had enough to eat. In our ancestors, this resulted in a balance wherein they were blessed with adequate reserves for emergencies, but not excess fat that could compromise their normal cell chemistry and make them sick.

The difference today is that we are no longer eating in ways that are consistent with our design. Food is available all day every day, and it is nutrient deficient, packed with calories, and very low in fiber. We consume only 10 percent of the fiber that was in our traditional, natural-food diet. Eating foods with less nutrition and fiber and more calories fools our appetite controls and results in our eating more and gaining weight. Today, 20 percent of our calories come from sodas with no nutrition or fiber. Most people consume high-fat animal products concentrated with calories, which again have no fiber to shut off the appetite. Wild-game meat contains up to 15 percent fat, while today's high-fat foods may be up to 80 percent fat, and fat has more than twice the calories as the same amount of carbohydrates. Because of the kinds of food we are eating—high-calorie, nutrient-deficient, fiberless, toxic, processed junk—the weight-gaining effects of gorging ourselves are enormously magnified. What would happen if we did not live this way? What if we were to return to eating a diet that was consistent with our design and contained fresh fruits, vegetables, whole grains, beans, nuts, and seeds?

Secrets of Aging with Vitality

The Hunzas, Vilcabambas, and Titicacas lived in remote mountainous regions of the Himalayas and Andes, isolated from the modern world. They were farmers who ate good diets, got plenty of exercise, and led low-stress lives. Only a century ago, they normally lived well into their hundreds, vigorous, fully functional, and free of disease. Among the Hunza people, men from teenagers to 120 years old performed physically demanding folk dances. Men in their seventies and eighties were observed gliding through the air with the same grace and ease as those in their teens and twenties. These people were unsurpassed in perfection of physique, and diseases such as cancer, heart disease, hypertension, diabetes, Alzheimer's, osteoporosis, and arthritis were totally unknown. Most never suffered even a cold, and they were never overweight, because they were healthy. Obesity is virtually unknown among tribal cultures eating traditional diets.

Even today, hundreds of thousands of people in their eighties and nineties enjoy superior health and happy, vigorous lives. These people are free of the chronic diseases that affect most of us, and they are never overweight. Where are these extraordinary people? Rural China. The United Nations refers to certain areas of China as "longevity-dense areas."

What is the secret of all these healthy, long-lived, and slender people? The secret is in their diet. They eat healthy, plant-based whole foods and engage in regular physical activity. Do they ever become overweight and develop the chronic diseases we suffer? Yes—when they start eating the toxic, nutritionally deficient, high-calorie processed foods that we eat.

Starving to Death While Getting Fat

Overweight is primarily a disease of malnutrition, with toxicity an important contributor. Deficiency alone can cause overweight. Dr. Michael Zemel of the University of Tennessee Nutrition Institute and other researchers have found that calcium deficiency can turn on fat-storing genes, while adequate calcium speeds fat burning. Similarly, a deficiency of omega-3 fatty acids activates fat-storing genes, while adequate omega-3s turn them off and speed up fat burning. So guess what? Most Americans are deficient in both calcium and omega-3s. All nutrients act synergistically as a team, yet the average American gets only a fraction of the nutrition they require for optimal health. We are thus operating at far below our biological potential, resulting in our epidemic of chronic disease and overweight. As long as the body is not getting the nutrition it needs, you will crave food even though you have just loaded up on high-calorie junk food.

A nutrient is a substance the body must obtain from outside itself in order to stay alive. No one food contains all the nutrients we need, and every person has unique nutritional needs. We must eat a variety of foods—the larger the variety, the better. Hardly any American is getting all the nutrients he or she needs on a daily basis. Estimates in medical journals run as high as 92 percent of Americans being deficient in one or more essential vitamins and minerals. The amount of fresh fruits and vegetables consumed by Americans has been declining for decades—not to mention that the nutritional content of fruits and vegetables has also declined, making a bad situation even worse.

From 1970 to 1994, caloric intake in the United States increased by 15 percent, while physical activity decreased. Most of the caloric increase was due to the increased consumption of nutritionally worthless sodas and junk foods. According to the Centers for Disease Control, average calorie consumption from carbohydrates alone increased by 300 calories per day between 1971 and 2000. Consuming these empty calories causes nutritional deficiencies, leading to disease of every description, including overweight.

As you seek to lose weight by consuming fewer calories and increasing exercise, you must make sure the calories you do consume are loaded with nutrition. You cannot simply eat smaller amounts of nutritionally worthless foods. You need to eat organic, fresh, raw fruits and vegetables, sprouts, beans, and whole grains—foods that contain the highest amount of nutrients and fiber per calorie. Because these real foods are both nutrient-rich and fiber-rich, they will make you feel fuller. This satisfies hunger, shuts off the appetite, and prevents the consumption of too many calories. Empty-calorie, nutrient-poor, fiberless, make-believe foods such as sugar, white flour, and most processed and fast foods are not options. They simply do not contain the nutrients required to keep you young and healthy by building healthy new cells to replace worn-out cells.

You might be asking, "What if I made the effort, changed my diet, and ate more whole, natural foods? Would I really lose weight?" Let us share our observations with you. In our experience, people who shift to a whole, natural-food diet lose an average of five to ten pounds per month until they reach their normal weight. Further, as long as they remain on such a diet, they do not gain that weight back. It's worth making the effort.

Toxins Make You Sick—and Fatter

Toxins in our food and in our environment play an important role in our overweight epidemic by distorting the body's ability to control both appetite and weight. Common food additives such as MSG and aspartame can make us feel hungry even when we do not need food. Chemicals used in common plastics such as phthalates and bisphenol A, as well as PCBs and solvents, are also associated with weight gain.

Animals exposed to pesticides can experience huge weight gains without any increase in caloric intake. Domesticated animals are fed growth promoters to fatten them up, but when you eat their meat you ingest those growth promoters, and they fatten you up. Even prescription drugs, including antihistamines, antidepressants, anti-inflammatories, and hormones, can cause weight gain.

The effects of toxins are magnified when poor diets deprive us of the essential nutrients that our detoxification systems need in order to remove toxins from our bodies. A major source of dietary toxins is processed junk food. Processed foods, from breakfast cereals to hot dogs to dinner helpers, are loaded with toxic artificial preservatives, colorings, and flavorings, plus nitrites, MSG, artificial sweeteners, and many other toxins. As toxins accumulate in our bodies, normal cell function is increasingly impaired, and premature aging along with health problems of every description, including overweight, result.

Fighting Fat as a Disease

All of us started life as a single cell, the smallest unit of life in the plant and animal kingdom. A mature body is made up of between 50 and 100 trillion such cells. Each cell is an individual unit of life that is part of a community—trillions of cells communicating and cooperating with each other. When our cells are healthy and functioning normally, the entire community functions harmoniously. When this happens, we say the body is in *homeostasis,* meaning that our body is in balance and able to function at its highest potential. *Health is the state in which all cells are functioning optimally, communicating and cooperating with each other, and the body is self-repairing, self-regulating, and balanced.* Being overweight is a diseased state where there is massive cellular malfunction resulting in injured molecules and cells, oxidized fats, cross-linked proteins, nutrient deficiencies, depleted enzymes, and metabolic chaos in general. In most cases, dieting only makes this situation worse.

No matter what name you give to a disease, *the essence of disease is that a massive number of cells are no longer functioning normally; they are no longer properly communicating, self-regulating, and self-repairing.* Getting well or losing weight permanently requires that this be reversed. When a person's cells are no longer operating normally, it can manifest as a common cold, the flu, polio, heart disease, arthritis, osteoporosis, diabetes, cancer, depression, or any other so-called disease, including overweight. The thousands of diseases that conventionally trained physicians categorize, diagnose, and treat are truly only one disease, which takes on many different faces because there are many thousands of possible combinations of cellular deficiencies and toxicities, all acting through a unique set of genes. These combinations produce a myriad of symptoms, giving the deceptive appearance of many diseases with unknown and mysterious causes.

Deficiency, one of the two causes of disease, frequently manifests as disease in certain organs because specific tissues require higher amounts of certain nutrients, and that amount is not being supplied in the diet. For example, both the prostate gland and the retina are zinc-rich tissues, requiring more zinc than other tissues. The thyroid gland is rich in iodine, and the female cervix rich in vitamin C and folate. When any nutrient is in short supply, the cells with the highest need are the first to suffer impaired function and show signs of distress. A deficiency of even one amino acid in the brain impairs thinking and behavior. The problems caused by these deficiencies create the illusion of different diseases with unknown causes—prostate enlargement, cervical cancer, thyroid impairment, mental and emotional problems, and so forth, yet all these "diseases" can result from a deficiency of a single nutrient that is required in larger than normal amounts by that specific tissue.

A zinc deficiency, for example, can cause cellular malfunctions manifesting as numerous so-called diseases, such as vision problems, including macular degeneration; skin problems, including acne; emotional problems; problems with attention span, learning ability, and short-term memory; enlarged prostate; immune suppression; and birth defects. Each individual has unique nutritional needs, and some people have exceptionally high needs for specific nutrients. In each case it will be the "limiting nutrient," the one that is in shortest supply, that determines the symptoms and the nature of the so-called disease produced. Zinc deficiency is common and is often a limiting nutrient. According to the USDA Continuing Survey of Food Intakes by Individuals (CSFII), zinc deficiency is a significant public health problem; 73 percent of Americans are not getting the recommended dietary amount of zinc mostly because modern farming methods have stripped the zinc out of our soils and therefore out of the foods.

Toxicity is the other cause of disease, and mercury toxicity is another significant public health problem. Most of the mercury we're exposed to comes from mercury-amalgam dental fillings, vaccinations, and fish. Some of the symptoms associated with mercury toxicity are depression, anxiety, hypertension, fatigue, irregular heartbeat, osteoporosis, allergies, asthma, sinus problems, rheumatoid arthritis, fibromyalgia, headaches, insomnia, and constipation. Mercury toxicity can produce asthma, depression, arthritis, high blood pressure, and osteoporosis—in the same person! That person may be seeing five different specialists who, almost certainly, never think of looking for the single cause. Rather, each specialist suppresses the different symptoms by prescribing a variety of toxic drugs. Unfortunately, the drugs increase the patient's toxic load, add to cellular malfunction, and create even more disease. Then we blithely call these new diseases "side effects," so as not to alarm people that they are now sicker than before.

Given the number of "diseases" that can be caused by just one deficiency or toxicity, such as zinc or mercury, imagine what might happen when multiple deficiencies and toxicities are working together at the same time. Unfortunately, most Americans are in this state. We suffer from combinations of deficiencies and toxicities that throw the body into biochemical chaos, producing a multitude of symptoms that baffle our physicians and cause them to mistakenly believe there are thousands of diseases. To modern medicine, disease is just one great big mystery!

Modern medicine embraces the idea that exposure to microorganisms will result in sickness. This is a myth. In order for infection to occur, your cells must already be malfunctioning and your immune system compromised. If this were not the case, everyone who is exposed to a particular pathogen would become sick. We know this does not happen.

An allergic reaction, eating sugar, a deficiency of vitamin C or zinc, lack of sleep, lack of exercise, stress, and many other factors impair immunity and allow you to become infected. You didn't "catch" that cold; you gave it to yourself by compromising your immunity. Healthy cells keep our immunity strong and hold infections at bay. Because they were healthy, people like the Hunzas lived to an average age of 120, without suffering as much as a cold. *You are not a powerless victim!* Because of the way we have been programmed to think about disease, this is probably a startling new thought.

Fortunately, cells have the ability to heal and repair, and the body is constantly replacing old, damaged cells with new ones. About 90 percent are replaced each year, so almost any disease, including overweight, can be reversed. The cells in the lining of our stomach are replaced every 2 days, liver and skin cells every 90 days, and blood cells every 120 days. If you are overweight or sick, the way to restore normal weight and health is to replace old, sick cells with healthy new cells. Once you understand this simple yet revolutionary concept, *you literally have the power to rebuild your body and prevent and reverse almost all disease.*

Are You Headed Toward Health or Premature Death?

Moving in the wrong direction toward cellular malfunction and weight gain can happen so slowly that we don't notice at first. The decline begins with a small number of cells malfunctioning, and slowly the number of unhealthy cells increases. By the time a disease is diagnosable, you have most likely been sick for a long time. Consider:

- Disease does not just randomly "happen," as many think.
- Overweight and other health problems are not inevitable results of aging.
- Health, not disease, is our natural state.
- Normal weight is the inevitable result of good health.

Our health is constantly changing along a continuum, varying as a result of the choices we make. Optimal health is at one end of the continuum, always accompanied by healthy weight. Death is at the other end, often accompanied by excess weight. Very few Americans are even close to the optimal health end of the continuum.

Between optimal health and death is pathology or diagnosable disease. Unfortunately, more than three out of four Americans have a diagnosable disease. Pathology is the point at which health has been seriously compromised, and cellular malfunction is occurring on such a large scale that the symptoms of a medically diagnosable disease are present. As the body becomes increasingly impaired by toxins and depleted of nutrient reserves, cellular damage begins to exceed daily repairs, and the body starts to age and fall apart. The body becomes less able to respond to new challenges, whether a pregnancy, a night out on the town, a long trip, a stressful experience, or exposure to toxic chemicals and infectious microorganisms. With reduced reserves, each new stress throws the system further out of balance. Finally, death is the state where all cells have ceased to function.

The Health and Disease Continuum

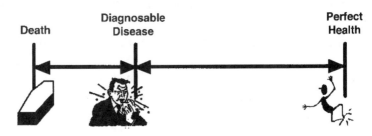

©2002 *Beyond Health*

Happily, your position on this continuum is not permanent. No matter how old or overweight you are, changing your direction is possible. We have personally witnessed miraculous turnarounds in individuals in their nineties, and even among advanced-stage cancer patients who initially appeared to be beyond hope. The human body is self-healing when we give it high-quality nutrition and stop giving it deadly toxins.

A lot of people we talk to mistakenly think they eat a good diet, even if it isn't perfect. What most people think of as a "good diet" will not prevent disease or restore health. Only a diet rich in nutrient-packed plant foods, along with high-quality supplements for insurance, supplies cells with the required raw materials to make all the necessary proteins, hormones, neurotransmitters, enzymes, antioxidants, and other chemicals they must have to solve our disease and weight problems and keep healthy.

Human health, and where you are and in what direction you are moving on the health and disease continuum, depends on the complex interaction of many factors. To help you understand and address these factors in a meaningful way, we offer the Six Pathways as weapons for you to employ in fighting fat. Each of these will be incorporated in your arsenal as you live the *NBFA* Lifestyle. Even if you focus on one pathway per week, in six weeks your body, mind, and spirit will be turning toward health and away from disease and overweight.

1. **Nutrition:** We live in the most-fed nation on Earth, which, ironically, is suffering from massive malnutrition. Ninety cents of the average food dollar is spent on processed foods that are low in nutrients and fiber but high in toxins and calories. You must learn how to empower your body with new food choices.

2. **Toxin:** Our accumulated burden of toxins is slowly destroying our health and contributing to our epidemic of chronic disease and overweight. Toxins are all around us, and many are unavoidable, which is why it is so important to avoid the toxins over which we do have control—in our homes, our food, and our personal-care products.

3. **Mental:** Your mind and body have an intricate connection so that thoughts play a role in weight control. Emotional stress can deplete your body of certain nutrients needed to metabolize fat and control appetite. You must learn to picture yourself in excellent health, vigorous physical condition, and at an ideal weight.

4. **Physical:** Lack of physical activity is a significant contributor to all disease, especially overweight. Regular exercise is not only necessary for weight reduction, it is critical for maintaining weight loss. Exercise resets the body's metabolism (the total of all the chemical reactions in your body) so that it burns more fat. It is also essential to deal proactively with stress, to have adequate rest, breathe fresh air, and get sufficient sunlight.

5. **Genetic:** Recent scientific advances have allowed us to understand how our diet influences our genes. Genes play a role both in our health and our size, but not the determining role that many believe. Obesity runs in families, but so do diet and lifestyle habits that give instructions to genes and contribute to obesity. Overweight families tend to have overweight pets, who certainly do not share their owner's genes. Genes do not and cannot explain the explosion in excess weight over the last several decades. Anyone can learn to optimize the expression of their genes through proper diet and lifestyle.

6. **Medical:** Modern medicine has become a "cut and drug industry" relying almost wholly on surgery and toxic chemicals to treat disease, including overweight. Rather than solving the problem of cellular malfunction, drugs make matters worse by causing more deficiency, toxicity, and disease. You must learn how to make your own researched decisions about which medical treatments to choose or reject.

Learning from Melissa's Success

Learning how to correct her deficient and toxic eating habits is what enabled Melissa, who we met earlier in this chapter, to regain her health. Melissa was able to lose weight, reverse aging, and eliminate fatigue and untreatable depres-

sion. In a year and a half, Melissa underwent a stunning transformation to vitality and joyful living. It was as though she
had been reborn.

Melissa had been overweight, sick, chronically tired, and
depressed her entire adult life. Rather than enjoying her life,
she was simply enduring it. For thirty years she had tried
numerous popular diet programs, but they provided only temporary weight loss followed by weight gain. Her gallbladder
had been surgically removed; she was prediabetic with high
blood sugar and triglycerides, and she suffered from one cold
after another along with insomnia, poor digestion, unhealthy
skin, and thinning hair. Her decades-long battle with depression had taken her from one doctor to another, leading to a
series of prescription drugs. Some provided temporary relief,
while others made her feel worse. All the while she continued
to gain weight. The combination of her chronic fatigue,
depression, and obesity made getting out of bed an ordeal. At
times, she felt suicidal.

Melissa often read books about weight loss, but she never
found them particularly helpful. She reported that when she
read *Never Be Sick Again* she felt for the first time she had
found something that made sense. She came to realize that all
of her problems, including her obesity and depression, were
the result of cellular malfunctions with common causes. She
began to reverse those malfunctions by addressing their
causes, thereby improving her cellular health. She began living the *Never Be Fat Again* Lifestyle, and in a matter of weeks
she noticed that she was not only feeling better, she was also
losing weight.

Melissa had grown up in a typical middle-American community. As an infant, she had been bottle-fed, which alone left
her vulnerable to a number of health problems. Cow's milk is
a particularly allergenic food, and Melissa's early exposure to
cow's milk resulted in a milk allergy. Fed a typical American
high-dairy diet, this allergy put a chronic load on her immune

system. Her overworked immune system caused her to succumb to one infection after another and to develop even more allergies. She was fed a meat-and-potatoes diet with lots of ice cream, cookies, cakes, and pies. Her diet lacked sufficient fresh fruits and vegetables, resulting in nutritional deficiency, and it contained a lot of toxins from the meat and dairy she was consuming. It also included excessive amounts of the deadly metabolic poison known as sugar, resulting in severely disturbed biochemistry and a destructive sugar addiction.

As an adult, Melissa took a high-pressure job in sales and eventually was involved in a difficult divorce, putting enormous stress on an already overtaxed system. Because she had grown up on a farm, she had been exposed to toxic agricultural chemicals. The human body is resilient, but it can only endure so much. A combination of poor nutrition, toxic exposures, lack of exercise, allergies, and chronic stress can and will do you in.

For most of her forty-eight years, Melissa had been headed in the wrong direction on the Six Pathways. From the Standard American Diet of her childhood, Melissa had progressed to low-fat (usually high-carbohydrate and almost always toxin-loaded) diet foods, splurging from time to time on sugary treats from an expensive health food store, which she mistakenly believed were healthier than similar treats from a regular supermarket. From her childhood exposure to agricultural chemicals, she had graduated to living in a congested urban environment with little consciousness that the toxins in this environment and in her home and body-care products could affect her health or weight.

On the Mental Pathway, Melissa's low self-esteem had led her into a stressful job where she constantly tried but failed to prove her worth, and then into a failed marriage. She never felt she had time for exercise, and she relied on diet drugs and antidepressants to get her through the day. Genetically, her family disposition toward allergies and overweight took their toll without a conscious and proactive response on her part.

After eighteen months on the *NBFA* Lifestyle, she went from being one hundred pounds overweight to having a slim, youthful figure. She looked radiant and appeared to be fifteen to twenty years younger than her chronological age. Her depression and fatigue were gone; she was bright and cheerful. She had so much energy she could outpace her twenty-six-year-old son. Her skin had become smooth and almost wrinkle free. Her hair had stopped falling out and looked full and beautiful. Her muscles were toned. It almost sounds impossible, doesn't it? But it's not. Melissa simply worked to improve her health rather than focusing on trying to lose weight.

Melissa began by avoiding the deadly "Big Four" (sugar, white flour, processed oils, and dairy/excess animal protein) and eating more fresh fruits, vegetables, whole grains, and a small amount of fish on occasion, plus incorporating high-quality nutritional supplements. With previous diets, Melissa always felt deprived. Now she didn't have to count calories. All she had to do was to eat fresh, unprocessed food as nature provides (that is, nutrient-rich foods)—as much of it as she liked! Trying to control her weight by eating less had never worked. When eating real food, she could satiate her appetite and still be on a low-calorie diet.

A good diet was only the foundation of her new lifestyle. For exercise, Melissa started rebounding on a high-quality mini-trampoline. She got rid of flab and started building muscle. She lowered her toxic load by avoiding processed foods; choosing different brands of toothpaste, shampoo, deodorant, skin creams, and household cleaning products; and purchasing filters for her shower, drinking water, and bedroom air. Upon discovering her sugar addiction, she broke it with nutritional supplements and dietary changes. A breakthrough occurred when we determined she had an allergy to gluten, a protein found in wheat and certain other grains. Melissa completely eliminated all wheat, rye, barley, and processed foods in order to avoid gluten. Once she removed gluten from her diet, the untreatable depression she had endured for thirty years disappeared.

Melissa's understanding of the concept of one disease expressing with many symptoms transformed her way of living. She no longer needed a different medical specialist for each disease. All she needed was the understanding that all of her diseases had common causes, which she, on her own, could reverse. She realized that her many health problems had the same two causes—deficiency and toxicity—that she had the power to change. A victim no longer, by managing her appetite and metabolism, she took charge, made better choices, and gained control over her life.

Your Body Fat Is Alive . . . and Deadly

Most people think of fat as a storehouse of unused calories. Far from it! Fat is biologically active, and recent research has found that not all fat is the same. Visceral fat, the type of fat found around your middle, is particularly deadly, which is why expanding waistlines are so dangerous. This type of fat invades internal organs and produces a flood of powerful chemicals that cause a wide range of problems including increased insulin, appetite, triglycerides, and blood pressure, resulting in heart disease, stroke, diabetes, arthritis, cancer, and premature death.

Excess fat throws much of the body's self-balancing into chaos, producing a cascade of health-damaging effects. Stored fat's biological activity results in the production of a variety of damaging chemicals, including hormones and inflammatory chemicals. The more fat you have, the worse it gets. Even being within normal weight guidelines may still be too fat. A 1987 study in the *Journal of the American Medical Association* found that the people who lived the longest weighed at least 10 percent below the numbers listed in the average body-weight tables.

Fat cells produce the hormone estrogen. Excess estrogen produced by fat cells throws the hormonal system, and then the entire body, out of balance. Excess estrogen is known to increase the risk of blood clots and heart attack, depress thyroid function, and promote skin, breast, and prostate cancer.

Fat cells produce a flood of dangerous inflammatory chemicals (including TNF-alpha and interleukin-6) which cause chronic systemic inflammation, resulting in free-radical damage to genes, cells, and tissues. These inflammatory chemicals age us, cause pain, and do most of the damage attributed to heart disease, diabetes, cancer, arthritis, Alzheimer's disease, and other health problems. They also interfere with fat storage controls, causing the body to store more fat, which then produces even more inflammation, causing the body to store even more fat in a vicious cycle.

Fat cells produce high levels of chemicals known to promote atherosclerotic plaque that clogs arteries. These chemicals interfere with insulin signaling, thus creating insulin resistance and type 2 diabetes. They interfere with the transport of key ions, such as potassium, across cell membranes, causing cells to malfunction. These same chemicals cause the secretion of hormones that constrict arteries and raise blood pressure. As you can see, fat doesn't just stare back at you in the mirror.

In addition, fat causes us to age rapidly. A June 2005 study in the medical journal *Lancet* found that being overweight accelerated aging by damaging chromosomes. Cells are damaged until they can no longer divide, thus shortening your life. The study concluded that, genetically speaking, obese women were almost nine years older than women of normal weight. Overweight people become biologically older faster.

Life Expectancy Is About to Decline

For the last two hundred years, average life expectancy in the United States has steadily increased, but according to a March 2005 study in the *New England Journal of Medicine,* that is about to change. Today's children and teens are so fat and so sick that, as they age, two to five years may be slashed from the current average U.S. lifespan of 77.6 years, the first reversal since the early 1800s.

More than one out of three children are overweight, and half of them are in the obese category. Because overweight people are more likely to get sick at younger ages and suffer more years of disability and poor health, today's overweight children face decreasing life expectancy due to a lifetime of more disease. Seventy-five percent of overweight children will go on to become overweight adults. As they grow older, these overweight children will suffer more heart disease, cancer, stroke, and other ailments. It boggles the mind to think that today we are seeing thirty-year-olds with the biological markers of eighty-year-olds. Imagine what is going to happen to these people as they age. They are going to add an unbearable burden to a healthcare system already in crisis.

Bad enough at present levels, the problem is projected to get worse. A 2006 study in the *International Journal of Pediatric Obesity* predicts that half of our children will be overweight by 2010. Overweight children develop up to five times as many fat cells as normal children. Because the number of fat cells cannot be decreased, maintaining normal weight becomes very difficult because the excessive number of fat cells limits how much weight can be lost.

Light at the End of the Tunnel

You can get well again by making a commitment to change your eating and living habits. This book teaches you how. The *NBFA* Lifestyle does not tell you what to eat and in what amounts. What it does is empower you with the knowledge to choose your own diet, one that suits you. The key is to improve the quality of your food and your lifestyle choices— eating a variety of nutrient-rich, fresh, whole-plant foods and arming yourself with effective weapons along the other five pathways. Your new, beautiful, strong, and lean body will mirror the good health that will be yours to enjoy for a lifetime. The *NBFA* Lifestyle works *if you work it!*

PART II

Eating the *NBFA* Way

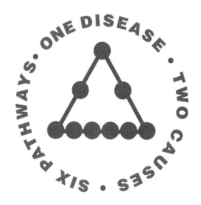

What you eat and avoid eating plays a major role in determining how your cells are nourished. Since nutrition is one of the six weapons you will use to triumph for good over excess pounds, this section contains valuable assistance. You learn that there are four major enemies of health and weight loss: the Big Four. The Big Four hide in many common foods, sabotaging your efforts to be healthy and slim. Other pieces of the nutrition puzzle and the effects of fast foods and processed foods are addressed. You learn about many foods that optimize cellular function and how to incorporate them into your meals to fight the battle for you.

AVOID 2 SUGAR

The Big Four are introduced in this chapter, revealing your enemies. The remainder of the chapter deals with the first of the Big Four: sugar. You will learn how sugar devastates cell chemistry, leading to compromised immunity and all manner of disease, not least of which is overweight. Among other information, you'll learn in this chapter:

- How sugar devastates your health and consequently your weight by creating biochemical chaos.
- How sugar robs the body of minerals.
- Why sugar accelerates the aging process.
- All the names by which sugar hides in your foods and which foods that you don't suspect actually contain sugar.
- How to substitute for sugar and learn why artificial sweeteners are not a good option.
- Even natural sugar in fruit can be an enemy if it is overeaten.

- Sugar is addictive, and withdrawal may be accompanied by symptoms.
- Practical ways to eliminate sugar.

Most of us are so accustomed to eating only what we like that the idea of eating for health comes as a shock.

—Russell L. Blaylock
Natural Strategies for Cancer Patients

Do you begin your busy day with coffee, cream, and Sweet'N Low or Equal, and a bowl of your favorite cereal? Pick up chicken fingers or a deli sandwich for lunch? Order a lean steak with a baked potato and sour cream for supper? Top off your day with chocolate cake or low-fat/sugar-free ice cream for dessert? These foods are our comfort foods. They are an integral part of most of our lives, but the diet just described—perhaps delicious and filling—is actually dangerous and inevitably causes disease, including overweight.

So many of these foods look good, taste good, and appear to be healthy that it is not always clear how deadly they are. They may be packaged in tantalizing ways, including words that make you think you are eating well. What is wrong with all these foods is that they contain what we call the Big Four: sugar, white flour, processed oils, and dairy/excess animal protein. Too much of the American diet consists of the Big Four, which is why the American diet is guaranteed to cause disease. This diet makes you sick and overweight because your body is deprived of critical nutrients, causing your appetite and weight-control systems to malfunction. A diet comprising the Big Four fills you up and fattens you up, but leaves you malnourished.

Meet Your Enemies: The Big Four

At least one and usually several of the Big Four can be found in almost all processed and fast foods. An essential part of the Nutrition Pathway of the *NBFA* Lifestyle involves eliminating these four danger foods:

1. sugar
2. white flour
3. processed oils
4. dairy/excess animal protein

This list may shock you because most people eat these ingredients every day. If this is what everyone eats, how can it be bad? And how bad can it be? The answer is: *bad enough for three out of four of us to have a diagnosable chronic disease, for cancer and heart disease to be epidemics, and for two out of three of us to be overweight!*

Sugar, by all of its names, appears in countless processed food items, even those not considered sweet. White flour is a staple in many processed foods, from breads, buns, muffins, and pastries to breakfast cereals, crackers, baking mixes, and pizzas; it shows up in nearly all meals. Hydrogenated and other processed oils are found in most commercial foods, as well as in your kitchen. Dairy products have been falsely advertised as healthy for bones and weight loss. Excess animal protein, in the form of cheese, eggs, processed meat, and other animal products, has become a major part of our diet. An inventory of your pantry and refrigerator will show just how prevalent these toxic, cancer-promoting, calorie-laden foods have become.

Most people, even when dieting, live on supermarket food, which is mostly make-believe food. It looks like food, most people believe it is food, but it does not meet the needs of our cells like "real" food. Real food is organically produced, fresh, whole, and unprocessed as nature provides; it contains the nutrients that nature intended. Real food includes fresh fruits, vegetables, legumes, sprouts, raw nuts, seeds, and whole grains in their unadulterated state. Only these foods supply cells with the critical nutrients they need. Understandably, in our society it is not easy to eat real food 100 percent of the time, but any effort to add more real food to your diet moves you toward health and away from disease and overweight.

Another damaging aspect of the Big Four diet is that it lacks fiber. Most people don't realize that fiber is an essential nutrient. Fiber helps to prevent disease and control appetite and weight, yet most people are dangerously deficient in fiber. Fiber fills the stomach, signals the brain that you are full, and shuts down your appetite. When you eat low-quality processed foods, lacking in nutrition and fiber, the brain keeps the appetite turned on. You consume more calories, which drives cholesterol and estrogen levels higher, and estrogen promotes skin, breast, and prostate cancers. According to World Health Organization statistics, 93 percent of the calories consumed by Americans consist of fiberless animal protein, processed oils, and refined carbohydrates. Processing wheat into white flour destroys 78 percent of the fiber. Most people consume a mere 5 percent of their calories from fiber-rich fruits, vegetables, and legumes. According to the 1999–2000 National Health and Nutrition Examination Survey, sodas and sweet drinks, which supply no fiber and little or no nutrition, have become the largest source of calories in the American diet. Consider that a sixty-four-ounce Big Gulp drink sold at convenience stores contains about eight hundred calories. The sugar in just one soda a day can cause you to gain twelve to fifteen pounds in a year.

Because there is so much to say about the negative health and weight effects of sugar, we devote the remainder of this chapter to this first of the Big Four. The following chapter focuses on the other three, as well as processed and fast food.

Sugar Makes You Sick and Fat

Quitting sugar alone will go a long way toward keeping you slim, healthy, and young because sugar makes you fat, sick, and old. Sugar is such a big part of our lives, most people find it difficult to comprehend how truly toxic this deadly substance is. Sugar is one of the deadliest poisons we are exposed to on a daily basis, and it is highly addictive; eating sugar is death by installment. If sugar were introduced today as a new product, the FDA could not approve it. FDA approval requires that a product be proven safe, and sugar is dangerous. Every time you eat sugar, the effect on your body is like a fifty-car pileup on the freeway—toxic spills, wreckage, injuries, chaos. Permanent injury is done from which you will never recover. Sugar wreaks havoc on your DNA, immune system, hormone system, cardiovascular system, nervous system, and cellular health; it ages you. You must ask yourself how often you want to damage your body this way. How fast do you want to age?

Eating sugar in excess of what can be immediately burned causes it to be stored in the liver in the form of glucose (glycogen). Since the liver's capacity is limited, a daily intake of refined sugar soon causes the liver to exceed its ability to store sugar, and the excess glycogen is returned to the blood in the form of fatty acids. These are taken to every part of the body and stored as fat in the most inactive areas: the belly, the buttocks, the breasts, and the thighs.

Sugar is everywhere, and almost everyone eats it daily—even if they don't consume desserts. Because we all grew up with sweets, few realize that refined sugar is relatively new to our diet. White sugar, as we know it, was first introduced in 1812; it became widely available only in the twentieth century. In 1900, per capita refined sugar consumption in the United States was less than ten pounds per year. Today it is around 160 pounds. Most Americans now get about 20 percent of their calories from sugar (and some get a lot more), which creates a massive and continual disruption to their biochemistry. Eating even two teaspoons of sugar creates a wide range of deficiencies and toxicities for a period of six to eight hours, causing massive cellular malfunction.

Sugar is added to the majority of processed foods, but refined sugar is actually an *unfood*. An unfood robs you of nutrition. In order to be metabolized, sugar requires certain nutrients, such as B vitamins, calcium, magnesium, chromium, and zinc. In the refining process, these nutrients are lost. So where does the body get them? It robs your bones, teeth, and other tissues of essential vitamins and minerals in order to process the sugar you are eating. In *A History of Nutrition,* Elmer McCollum cites experiments in which animals fed water alone lived substantially longer than those fed sugar and water. In other words, *eating sugar is worse than eating nothing!*

Is Your Body in Chaos?

When we consume sodas or foods containing sugar, white flour, or other refined carbohydrates, blood sugar rapidly increases and a cascade of catastrophic biological events is triggered. Here are some of them.

Damaging Acidity

Sugar is acid forming in the body, and when consumed daily it produces a continuously over-acid condition, which is one of the common denominators of disease. Sugar is so rapidly absorbed into the bloodstream and quickly distributed to body cells that there is insufficient oxygen available to effectively burn and metabolize the sugar. The result of this incomplete burning is the formation of excess pyruvic acid, which has a toxic effect on the body. When the body becomes acidic, precious minerals, such as calcium, are lost from the bones and teeth as the body tries to neutralize the acid and rectify the imbalance. This acidic condition fundamentally changes your body chemistry and causes disease such as osteoporosis. Cancer thrives in an acidic environment. Further, pyruvic acid accumulates in the brain and nervous system and damages these tissues, causing neurological disease and contributing to Alzheimer's disease.

Impaired Immunity

Sugar is a leading cause of infections. Sugar depresses immunity by interfering with vitamin C metabolism, leading to colds, flu, pneumonia, other infections, and even cancer. Immune cells need a lot of vitamin C to function normally. In fact, white blood cells require fifty times as much vitamin C inside the cell as outside. Sugar and vitamin C have a similar chemical structure and compete with one another to enter cells. When a lot of sugar is present, it wins the competition, creating an artificial shortage of vitamin C. Without adequate amounts of vitamin C, the immune system becomes severely compromised.

Another mechanism by which sugar damages immunity is by altering blood-sugar levels. Blood sugar must be kept within normal limits so that the amount of blood sugar and the amount of blood oxygen are in balance. When sugar is part of your diet, blood-sugar levels are changing constantly, bouncing between too high and too low, and cells can be deprived of critical oxygen, which damages cells and suppresses immunity. *Even a small amount of refined sugar suppresses your immune system.* Sugar promotes cancer both by depressing immunity and because cancer cells require more sugar than normal cells. Cancer patients should never eat sugar. Even natural sugar from fruits can feed cancer.

Mental Disorders

Sugar consumption figures prominently in emotional and psychological disorders. Sugar leads to imbalanced moods, poor concentration, phobias, obsessive-compulsive disorders, and depression. It is a key player in behavior disorders such as

ADD and ADHD for which we are drugging so many individuals, often innocent children. Many of the symptoms of
ADHD are remarkably similar to those of sugar sensitivity. In
Sugar Blues, William Dufty writes, "Today, pioneers of ortho-
molecular psychiatry [using nutrients to normalize brain func-
tion] . . . have confirmed that mental illness . . . and . . .
emotional disturbances can be merely the first symptom of the
obvious inability of the human system to handle the stress of
sugar dependency."

Excess Insulin

Eating sugar and refined carbohydrates causes a rapid and dangerous increase in blood sugar. The body responds to this crisis
by secreting insulin from the pancreas, causing an insulin spike.
Insulin signals cells to lower blood sugar. The cells absorb the
sugar, which is either burned for energy or stored as fat. However,
the creation of excess insulin creates a cascade of negative effects,
including diabetes, high blood pressure, heart disease, high
cholesterol, Alzheimer's disease, cancer, and, of course, overweight. Indeed, as long as insulin remains high, your cells retain
fat instead of burning it, and all the new fat you eat is stored.
*Insulin causes cells to store fat, and stored fat causes insulin to
increase, resulting in a vicious cycle of adding more fat.*

Excess insulin wreaks havoc in the following ways:

- Insulin signals cells to absorb excess sugar, which solves
the problem of too much sugar in the blood, but it creates
a host of new problems. Now the body's cells have too
much sugar. To correct this imbalance, cells turn the sugar
into saturated fat.

- Eating refined sugar or even too much natural sugar in
fruit juice is like eating saturated fat. This fat is stored
around your middle, in your blood vessels, and all over
your body, including your liver. You don't even have to be
overweight to have this harm you.

- Stored fat, even in small amounts, makes blood vessels less elastic, thus increasing risk of high blood pressure and cardiovascular disease. This effect also happens in children, making them more susceptible to cardiovascular disease as they age.

- Once in the blood, excess insulin remains elevated for hours, continuing to remove sugar from the blood, resulting in low blood sugar (hypoglycemia). As blood sugar drops below normal, appetite increases, and so we eat more sugar trying to restore normal blood sugar. This results in a vicious cycle of too much and too little blood sugar, causing chronically high insulin levels, sugar craving, and fat deposits.

- Low blood sugar starves the brain, which uses glucose almost exclusively for fuel. Starved of glucose, brain cells are unable to produce sufficient energy.

- Energy-deprived cells become more vulnerable to the damaging effects of chemicals called excitotoxins. Excitotoxic chemicals, such as MSG, are used as flavor enhancers in most processed foods. The damage caused by excitotoxins contributes to brain diseases such as Alzheimer's disease.

- Chronic high insulin levels contribute to diabetes by causing the fat content of cells to increase, making the cells less sensitive to insulin (insulin resistance).

- When cells are resistant to insulin's message, more insulin is required to do the same job. The body pumps out more insulin as it tries harder to lower blood sugar levels, resulting in both high blood sugar and insulin. Meanwhile, since the insulin can't do its job, cells are unable to obtain sufficient glucose.

- Without enough glucose, cells can't produce energy, and we become weak and fatigued, which disrupts normal metabolism, generating free radicals and damaging cells and DNA.

- Free radicals (highly reactive chemicals that attack

molecules crucial for cell function) cause inflammation, contributing to diseases of every description, including cancer, heart disease, autoimmune diseases, Alzheimer's disease, arthritis, osteoporosis, and diabetes. Even a modest increase in blood sugar generates a flood of free radicals, and this is why diabetics suffer so many serious complications.

- Insulin inhibits mobilization of previously stored fat, keeping it right where it is.
- Insulin stimulates our livers to produce cholesterol, resulting in high cholesterol.
- Insulin interferes with enzymes and inhibits the body's production of certain healthy, omega-3 fatty acids.
- As insulin levels rise, magnesium is depleted because magnesium is required to produce insulin. Lack of magnesium contributes to insulin resistance, thus increasing the need for insulin and lowering magnesium even more in a vicious cycle. Low magnesium causes blood vessels to constrict and blood pressure to go up.
- Sugar causes calcium and magnesium losses in the urine. As long as insulin levels stay high, it is very difficult to replace these mineral losses, thus contributing to osteoporosis. Even if you consume a lot of calcium, as long as insulin remains high, the calcium is not properly metabolized, leading to calcification of tissue, including in your arteries, and even the growth of calcified tumors.
- Insulin causes sodium retention, which causes retention of fluids, increasing weight. Fluid retention causes blood pressure to increase and other problems, such as congestive heart failure.
- Insulin stimulates the sympathetic nervous system, which can cause arteries to constrict or go into spasm. This can precipitate a heart attack in susceptible people, which is why some people are more prone to heart attacks after eating a high-carbohydrate meal.

- Insulin tells kidney cells to hold on to salt, which causes high blood pressure.
- Animal studies have shown that aging is largely controlled by insulin. People who live the longest eat the least sugar and have the lowest insulin.

Excess blood insulin is one of the most devastating things that can happen to you because it leads not only to overweight, but to heart disease, cancer, dementia, and inflammation throughout your body. Yet insulin spikes every time you eat sugar, and if you eat sugar several times a day, insulin remains high all day, every day. Some researchers even believe that insulin may be the single largest cause of chronic disease.

Hormones Wreak Havoc

Most Americans, both men and women, suffer from hormones that are out of whack, which substantially contributes to our chronic disease epidemic. To keep your body well regulated and in balance, all of your cells must constantly communicate with each other. Hormones are messenger molecules and a critical part of the body's communications system. Anything that disrupts hormones disrupts cellular communications, leading to disregulation and disease. Sugar throws your hormones (adrenaline, cortisol, thyroid, estrogen, and others) into chaos, contributing to imbalances and chronic diseases.

Hormone problems get worse when you consider that the fat in an overweight individual is not just extra padding. Fat cells are biologically active. They produce even more estrogen, adding to the excess that is already there and working to keep us overweight. Fat cells both store and release fats on an ongoing basis. When fat cells are under the influence of estrogen, they store more fat and release it less willingly. High estrogen levels make weight loss nearly impossible, and eating sugar increases insulin, which increases estrogen.

Alert: Sugar Hides in Unsuspected Foods

The chaos caused by eating sugar compels Nancy Appleton, author of *Lick the Sugar Habit,* to say that "sugar so upsets the body chemistry that it doesn't matter what else you put in your mouth; neither healthful food nor junk food will digest properly." With sugar in the system, our bodies cannot adequately process even high-quality foods. These undigested foods ferment and putrefy in the stomach and gut, creating dangerous toxins, which is why it is a bad idea to eat a hamburger and a cola, or a breakfast cereal containing sugar; the meat putrefies and the cereal ferments. Many people suffer indigestion after eating a meal with a sugary dessert, which impairs digestion.

Worthy of special mention is fructose, as many people believe it is safer because it is "fruit sugar." In truth, fructose may be even more dangerous to your health and weight than sucrose (table sugar), and it is everywhere in our diet, including sodas, jellies, pastries, hamburgers, ketchup, salad dressings, and corn syrup. Studies show that fructose disturbs levels of appetite-controlling hormones even more than sucrose, causing people to feel hungry and eat more. Fructose also causes long-lasting increases in triglycerides, which get stored as fat, increase insulin resistance and diabetes, and increase the risk of cardiovascular disease. If you feed fructose to laboratory animals, they rapidly become obese. Some researchers believe that high-fructose corn syrup found typically in soft drinks is the greatest contributor to the epidemic of obesity.

Getting sugar out of your diet is a simple choice that we can all make, but you may be surprised to learn how many processed foods you consume contain sugar. About eighty-five different forms of sugar are found in processed foods. Getting sugar out of your eating regimen means much more than eliminating desserts. You must learn to be a label reader. When you read labels, look for more than just the word *sugar* in the list of ingredients. Below is a partial list of some of the names that tell you sugar is in that product. Copy this list and carry it with you when you shop.

barley malt	high-fructose corn syrup
beet sugar	honey
brown rice syrup	lactose
brown sugar	malt syrup
cane sugar	maltodextrin
confectioner's sugar	maltose
corn syrup	maple syrup
dextrose	molasses
evaporated cane juice	organic sugar
fructose	raw sugar
fruit juice concentrate	sugar
fruit juices	sugar cane syrup
glucose	turbinado sugar

Notice how many of the words end in "ose." Words that end in "ose" (dextrose, fructose, glucose, maltose, etc.) are usually a form of sugar. Many product labels, even in health food stores, contain not just one of these items, but three or four. That adds up to a lot of insulin-producing, havoc-wreaking consequences. One good idea is to check the number of grams of sugar you may be consuming. *If it is more than four grams in the amount you intend to eat, reject the item.* Best of all is to reject any item with added sugar. Look at the ingredients on a can of baked beans, which is a processed food that should be avoided anyway. A typical can may read: white beans, water, molasses, sugar, fructose, brown sugar; this product is loaded with four different kinds of sugar. A typical can may contain 20 grams of sugar.

Here is another list to keep in mind: food products that, perhaps unexpectedly, contain sugar. This list can help you get started, but it is by no means exhaustive.

bacon
bacon bits
baked beans
BBQ sauces
bologna
boxed cereal (even healthy-
    looking ones)
bread
bullion cubes
canned fruit
canned soups
coffee creamers
crackers
croutons
cured meats
deli meats
dips
dried fruits
dry-roasted nuts
flavored coffees
granola
ham
hot dogs
ketchup
marinades
mayonnaise

pancake syrup
peanut butter
pepperoni
pickles
pizza sauce
prepared teas
processed meals
relish
salad dressing
salsas
salt (some brands)
sausage
seasoning mixes
smoked meats
soup starters
soy creamers
soy and rice milks
soy/tofu meat substitutes
spaghetti sauce
spice mixes
steak sauces
supplement bar/shake
trail mixes
vitamin waters
yogurt

All these items are processed. Stick with unprocessed whole foods, and you won't need to worry about added sugar. Fresh broccoli, sunflower sprouts, Brazil nuts, and brown rice don't have ingredient lists to worry about, and none of these have added sugars. Sugar improves the shelf life and flavor of processed foods and therefore is added to most of them. Fresh, whole foods simplify life.

As you avoid all of the sweeteners listed as sugars, you can use a little pure stevia extract when sweetness is necessary. Stevia is a naturally sweet, calorie-free herb. In fact, it is one hundred times sweeter than sugar. Stevia is not harmful like sugar, and furthermore is listed as one of twelve superfoods to transform your health by Dr. Gillian McKeith in her book,

Living Food for Health. Dr. McKeith, director of the McKeith Clinic in London and a highly respected clinical nutritionist, says, "Stevia has the ability to regulate blood-sugar levels, suppress sweet cravings, and lessen hunger pangs," adding that "it may be effective for those suffering from diabetes and hypoglycemia. Stevia is excellent for stimulating mental and physical stamina, and it can even suppress the bacteria that cause tooth decay."

Substitute with Care, and Beware

Once you have gotten the sugar out of your system and no longer crave it, occasional (but not daily) use of a small amount of pure raw honey as a treat is acceptable. There is some nutritional value in honey since the nutrients are not all stripped away. Beware, though, that supermarket honey is usually highly processed and often adulterated with other forms of sugar, such as corn syrup. Honey from a beekeeper is recommended. Choose raw honey since pasteurized honey has been heated, which destroys enzymes and nutrients necessary for its digestion. Raw honey is cloudy and an off-white color. If it is transparent, it is not raw.

Only after your sugar addiction is broken can less-refined sweeteners be consumed on infrequent and special occasions. These include organic blackstrap molasses, evaporated cane juice, or agave nectar. The less refined a sweetener is, the more acceptable. Less-refined sugars can be sneaky, though, creeping in to your diet slowly but increasingly. Never let it become a daily habit. Once a sugar addict, easily a sugar addict again.

We have seen many health seekers make a common mistake. They cut out sugar, but instantly began to substitute by using less-refined sweeteners, artificial sweeteners, or even natural sugar provided by fruit. Maintaining the same lifestyle with better sweeteners is not the best choice. These substitutes still cause your body to produce excess insulin and can create havoc just as sugar does. They do not result in the cellular health that is our goal. Health-food stores are loaded with items that are sweet, highly processed, and unhealthy. The main difference between them and their grocery-store counterparts is that they are considerably more expensive. Weight loss will not result from consuming these more expensive goodies in place of your old junk food. Reserve some treats (see chapter 13 for healthier desserts) for special occasions only, not daily consumption.

"Natural" Sugar Takes a Toll Too

The natural sugar in whole fruit is fine in moderation. Fruit eaten whole has a powerhouse of vital enzymes, vitamins, minerals, and phytochemicals, and it also has fiber, which helps to reduce the insulin response to the natural sugar. Eating fresh, organic fruit daily is a healthful practice and is highly recommended in the *NBFA* Lifestyle. Fruit should also be eaten alone or only when combined with certain foods, as discussed in the next chapter.

Fruit juice is another story. We do not recommend drinking fruit juice (even freshly juiced at home) or giving it to children because the lack of fiber allows for rapid absorption of its natural sugar, which can throw the body out of balance. Fruit juice is a poor food choice, yet processed apple juice makes up 50 percent of all fruit servings to preschool children. Sweetening foods with fruit juice concentrates (even worse than fruit juice) is not recommended for these same reasons.

If you have a strong sugar addiction, you may need to avoid fruits for a few weeks until your cravings subside. Limit your fruits to one or two pieces a day. Don't allow yourself to get in the habit of satisfying all of your sugar cravings with fruit; too much can imbalance you. If you decide to completely avoid fruit initially, add fruit back in slowly and cautiously, beginning with fruits that are not as sweet, such as apples, peaches, pears, and melons, once or twice a week. Eating a few soaked nuts with your fruit can moderate the resulting rise in blood sugar.

Don't lose heart. After a while, your taste buds will change. Naturally sweet foods will taste sweeter—not only fruits, but carrots, sweet potatoes, beets, tomatoes, and jicama. In time, sugar may even taste disgustingly sweet and unappealing. You will find you look forward to fruit and enjoy it as you never have before.

So many varieties of fruit exist that you don't need to get bored with the same five or six. Did you know that you could try a new fruit every day this year and still not try them all? Variety is critical to providing the full spectrum of antioxidants, vitamins, and minerals to your body. Try to get out of the rut of consuming the same two or three fruits week after week. You may even want to go to an Asian market, a fruit market, or online to find new and delicious options. When you travel, take advantage of the opportunity to discover different fruit that is indigenous to that area.

Expect Withdrawal Symptoms

Getting off refined sugar can be more difficult for some people than it is for others, depending upon your body chemistry and your former use of sugar. The fact is, sugar acts like a drug and is addictive, similar to alcohol, heroin, and other drugs. Most Americans have a sugar addiction, and only a handful realize it.

As we have described, a short time after eating sugar your blood sugar can drop below normal, and when this happens, cravings for more sugar begin. The more sugar you eat, the more sugar you will want. People begin to depend upon sugar for a quick pick-me-up. The first dose comes in a processed breakfast cereal; by midmorning another fix is needed. In time, your body becomes exhausted by the roller-coaster ride on sugar highs and lows, and it will no longer be able to regain balance. Health will then break down quickly.

What are the symptoms of withdrawal? They can vary, so each person will not experience all of these: dizziness, headaches, shakes, depression, anger, sweats, light-headedness, fatigue/lethargy, strong cravings (which can be almost overwhelming), irritability, and moodiness (unexpected changes from high to low). Most individuals can overcome these symptoms within several days to a week. Some people may choose to wean themselves off sugar gradually, but remember that this is not the most merciful way to treat yourself since eating a little sugar makes you crave more. The best course is to go cold turkey.

Diane, who was one of Raymond's clients, told how she and her husband had changed their diet and were feeling incredible; they were experiencing enormous energy, vitality, and health. All of this came to a crashing halt when one evening meal was topped off with a piece of wedding cake. Since Diane's mother-in-law was a bit embarrassed by her son and daughter-in-law's new health kick, she had requested that they attend a family wedding and eat as "normal" people do. Wanting to be nonoffensive, they decided to comply. Months later, Diane told me how that one dinner began their downward spiral, and how difficult it was to get back on track.

Taming the Sugar Monkey

We have been conditioned to associate food with comfort from our earliest days—from giving desserts to children to celebrating birthdays and holidays with sweets: birthday cake and ice cream, holiday cookies, and candies. As a result, changing your diet—in particular, eliminating sugar—can be an intensely emotional struggle. This section is full of suggestions to help you to break the emotional ties to sugar.

Keep a food journal (see appendix B and C for sample

pages that can be copied, increased to 8½ x 11 size, and put in a notebook). For long-term success in losing weight, continual self-monitoring is required, and food journals have proven to be one of the simplest and most effective tools. In fact, weight-loss experts agree that patients who are not ready to keep a diary may not be ready to lose weight. We recommend that you write down everything you eat and also track your cravings by recording when and in what circumstances they occur. Do they occur when you are under stress, depressed, or after you eat a certain type of food such as cooked starches? After a while you can ascertain which foods cause you to crave sweets. Stressful circumstances can cause the pancreas to secrete insulin, which may bring on sugar cravings. Recognizing such patterns will help you to overcome them. A nutrient-rich snack will go much further in helping your cells deal with stress or emotional lows than will nutrient-robbing sugar. Healthy proteins and fats will help to stabilize blood sugar fluctuations brought about by stress.

When sugar cravings hit, be ready with strategies to overcome them, such as making yourself wait for fifteen minutes to see if the craving will subside. During this time, imagine the guilt you will feel if you do indulge. Also imagine the positive triumph you will feel if you do not. Another strategy: when a craving comes, get your mind off of it by going out and exercising. Rebound on a mini-trampoline, dance, bike, or just take a walk. Physical activity helps dull the appetite. When you want to eat sugar, work on a hobby that requires both hands, such as piano, a craft project, or a favorite sport. You can't eat with both hands occupied.

The encouragement of a friend or family member who wants to give up sugar too is ideal. When you are craving sugar, call that person, and they can do the same. Tell coworkers, friends, and family members that you are getting off sugar for your health. The fact that you have shared your commitment with them may help you to stick to it in times of temptation, even if it is only out of pride at not wanting them to see you fail. Hopefully they will not offer you sugary foods if they know you are trying to quit.

Last, don't allow yourself to think that sugar will make you happy. It may bring enjoyment for the few moments that it is on your tongue, but those moments are fleeting, and the price you will pay for them is huge. Sugar will make you overweight, old, and sick. Contrary to making you happy, sugar usually leaves a person depressed, anxious, and moody. The real and lasting happiness comes when sugar is cut out: unwanted pounds melt away, health improves, you look and feel younger, and you know you have made the best choice. Be confident and think positively about what a beneficial change this will be for your health and the health of your family. Don't allow yourself to think negative, self-pitying thoughts about this change. Begin eating to *live*!

Here's How to Eliminate Sugar

- Keep sugar out of your house so it is not easily available. If you must go out to buy sugar in order to eat it, this will give you time to talk yourself out of it. The hassle of going out to buy it may also deter you.
- When you get a desire for sweets, drink a large glass of pure water. At times the body mistakes thirst for hunger, and drinking water at least fills your stomach temporarily.
- Have healthy snacks, such as a piece of fruit, raw nuts and seeds, or carrot and celery sticks, readily available.
- Cut salt from your diet, which helps you avoid sugar cravings. Salt and sugar are like opposites; when your body receives too much of one, it may crave the other, which is why a sugar binge can lead to a desire for chips, pretzels, or something salty (or vice versa).
- Do not eat corn or corn products. Many people with sugar addictions are also allergic to corn, whether they realize it or not. Much of the sugar in processed food is derived

from corn. Eating large quantities of sugar, over time, can cause a corn allergy, and the allergic reaction to corn can initiate a sugar craving. You must watch for and avoid not just corn, but corn syrup, cornstarch, cornmeal, tortilla chips, and all other forms of corn. Corn is often high in carcinogenic aflatoxins, toxins produced by mold on the corn, and almost all of the corn in the United States today, including organic corn, is contaminated with potentially harmful, genetically modified varieties.

- Avoid all caffeine, artificial sweeteners, and alcoholic drinks since they increase sugar cravings (especially in hypoglycemics—people with abnormally low blood sugar).
- Eat regular, balanced meals. Becoming extremely hungry sparks sugar cravings as the body seeks quick energy. This is especially important for hypoglycemic individuals. Six small meals a day can help a recovering hypoglycemic. Never skip breakfast.
- Eliminate white flour, white rice, and regular pasta, which turn to sugar once in the body, creating imbalances and sugar cravings. All processed carbohydrates trigger sugar cravings (more about this as we continue with the Big Four).
- If you know that you usually crave sugar after a meal, floss and brush your teeth immediately. The desire not to repeat the process may help to dissuade you from further eating.
- Being tired can precipitate sugar cravings. You have probably conditioned your body to turn to sugar for quick energy. Get plenty of good sleep.

If you should give in to a sugar craving, don't beat yourself up. Throw out any of the "poison" that remains. It is better in the trash than in your body. Get back on track. Make sure you record in your journal just how the sugar made you feel physically and emotionally so that you can read that the next time you face temptation. After eating the sugar, exercise to reduce its negative effects. Physical activity helps burn the sugar to prevent it from being stored as fat.

Some supplements are useful in reducing your desire for sugar. Chromium, manganese, and zinc are three minerals that help to regulate your blood-sugar levels. A good multivitamin contains adequate amounts of these nutrients in the right balance (see appendix D for suggestions). Vitamin C supplementation is also critical. Since vitamin C and sugar use the same biochemical pathway, supplementing with vitamin C helps to reduce sugar urges. The amino acid L-glutamine, found in many foods high in protein such as fish and beans as well as supplements, also helps to reduce sugar cravings. Three thousand milligrams per day in divided doses is usually sufficient; a quality glutamine supplement should also contain pyridoxal alpha-ketoglutarate (PAK) to help metabolize it more effectively (see appendix D for suggestions). Other supplements that help with cravings include gamma aminobutyric acid (GABA) and 5-hydroxytryptophan (5-HTP).

What About Artificial Sweeteners to Replace Sugar?

Artificial sweeteners can be just as addictive as sugar. Our society has made the mistake of seeking to cut calories and control sugar-related health problems (such as diabetes) by resorting to unnatural, synthetic chemicals, which create a whole new set of problems. It is a case of trading one poison for another equally, if not a more, dangerous poison. Artificial sweeteners are not an option in the *NBFA* Lifestyle. Processed foods, including Jell-O, ice cream, popsicles, baked goods, chewing gum, sodas, and many other so-called foods often fed to young children, typically contain artificial sweeteners. The answer to sugar-related health issues is to avoid both sugar and artificial sweeteners such as aspartame (NutraSweet), sucralose (Splenda), saccharin (Sweet'N Low), and others.

Information on the dangers of aspartame abounds. The FDA has far more complaints about aspartame than any other non-drug. Scientific data indicates that aspartame is metabolized in the body into a type of neurotoxin called an excitotoxin. Excitotoxins alter brain function, cause damage to the nervous system, and create systemic organ malfunction. (More information is available on the www.beyondhealth.com website, where you may access articles on aspartame and excitotoxins.)

Aspartame purports to be an aid to weight loss, but it often has the opposite effect. Research shows that one of the side effects of aspartame is carbohydrate cravings, which lead to weight gain, not loss. Many individuals have dropped ten or twenty pounds just by eliminating aspartame. Aspartame can be addictive, and the best way to deal with aspartame is to learn to live without it. The recipe section of this book gives you ideas for making tasty, healthy drinks with stevia to replace your diet drinks.

Saccharin has also been the topic of much research, and there is conclusive evidence about its dangers. While no longer on the government's list of cancer-causing substances, animal research indicates that saccharin increases appetite and causes an increase in food consumption, making the animals fat. In addition, when the sweet taste is not accompanied by the usual calories, the weight-control mechanisms may be disrupted, leading to less-efficient calorie burning and more weight gain

Sucralose (Splenda) is a more recent addition to the artificial sweetener market. Like aspartame, sucralose is an unnatural molecule, and no long-term studies have tested its safety. Sucralose is a man-made chemical synthesized by chlorinating sugar. The use of chlorine in this molecule is cause for concern, especially since the long-term effects of ingesting sucralose are unknown. This compound breaks down in the body into small amounts of 1,6-dichlorofructose, a chemical that has not been adequately tested in humans. Preliminary research indicates that sucralose can cause the thymus gland to shrink up to 40 percent. The thymus gland is a critical part of the immune system, helping to protect against infections. In addition to this disturbing news, sucralose was also found to cause enlarged livers and kidneys in early studies. Our advice is to avoid this sweetener.

If you need added incentive to subtract sugar, consider Heather's story. Heather came to Michelle for weight-loss guidance and began the *NBFA* Lifestyle by eliminating one of the Big Four each week for four consecutive weeks, while increasing consumption of fresh, raw vegetables, fruits, nuts, and seeds. During the first week, when she simply eliminated sugar (in all of its forms) and began eating more fresh raw produce, she lost six and a half pounds. Pam's experience is also inspiring. When Pam first approached Raymond, she was very resistant to changing her diet. After educating her regarding the dangers of sugar, she was willing to give up just sugar and alcohol. In six months she lost fifty pounds.

As you can see from this chapter, eating sugar increases oxidative free-radical damage in the body; stresses one's hormones; interferes with vitamin C transport; suppresses the immune system, causing infections; robs the body of minerals such as calcium, magnesium, chromium, potassium, and zinc; robs the body of vitamins, especially the Bs; accelerates aging; and creates biochemical havoc in general. If you do only one thing after reading this book—*cut sugar out of your life!*

AVOID WHITE FLOUR, PROCESSED OILS, DAIRY, AND EXCESS ANIMAL PROTEIN

This chapter rounds out the Big Four by revealing the truth about white flour, processed oils, dairy products, and excess animal protein. Among the information you'll learn in this chapter:

- How white flour robs your body of nutrients, what foods contain it, and how to live without it.
- What we mean by processed oil, why it is so harmful, and how to select good oils.
- Why today's meat is not even "real" meat, what makes it so harmful, how it stimulates weight gain, and why it is not needed for protein.

- How dairy products contribute to overweight and are not necessary for calcium intake.
- Why caffeine, though not one of the Big Four, can also be devastating to health and derail weight-loss efforts.
- How processed food sabotages healthy weight.
- Why fast food should be a crispy apple or a handful of raw Brazil nuts rather than more popular fast foods, which are devastating.

We have shown in experimental animals that cancer growth can be turned on and off by nutrition. . . . These findings are nothing short of spectacular.

—T. Colin Campbell
The China Study

Unfortunately, sugar is not the only prominent component of our diet that is causing overweight and disease. Cutting white flour, processed oils, dairy, and excess animal protein from your diet will greatly decrease your intake of processed and fast food and thus help you along the pathway to health.

White Flour—Sugar in Disguise

White flour, a staple in the Standard American Diet, is the second of the harmful Big Four and a major contributor to weight problems. Consuming white flour is essentially the same as eating sugar because the body quickly metabolizes it into sugar, thus causing the same problems that sugar does. Whether in the form of bread, pasta, buns, rolls, tortillas, pita pockets, pizza crust, crackers, croutons, breakfast cereal, pastries, donuts, cookies, cakes, pies, or some other convenience food, Americans consume an unbelievable average of 200 pounds of white flour per person per year. Add 200 pounds of this make-believe food to the 160 pounds of sugar we eat, and you have an annual consumption of 360 pounds per person of toxic, nutritionally worthless junk food.

Just like sugar, white flour is an antinutrient—an unfood. Almost all of the nutrients once contained in the wheat are intentionally removed with the bran or lost in the milling process, including 95 percent of the vitamin E, all of the essential fatty acids, and 78 percent of the vitamin B6. White flour is so depleted of nutrients that it robs the body of precious nutrient reserves in order to metabolize it. Very simply, eating white flour costs you more nutrients than you get. The result is nutrient deficiency that causes myriad health problems.

White flour has been associated with constipation, hemorrhoids, colitis, and rectal cancer because it is stripped of the fiber necessary to move it through the system. Ingredients such as "enriched wheat flour," "unbleached wheat flour," and "wheat flour" are merely different terms for wheat that has been processed into white flour. Because eating white flour raises blood sugar and insulin levels, your body is instructed to store fat. In June 2003, researchers at Tufts University reported that people who ate white bread gained three times as much weight as those who ate the same quantity of wholegrain bread. We don't recommend regular consumption of any bread. When grains are processed into flour to make bread, too many nutrients are lost.

Bread is not a healthy staple, and for an overweight person should be off limits. Even for those who are not overweight, bread is a poor choice because it is a processed food. As you forego white flour and look for other grains to use, keep in mind that wheat is a gluten-containing grain. Gluten is a protein in wheat, spelt, kamut, rye, barley, and oats (although there is some debate about oats). Symptoms may or may not be apparent, but up to half of the population may be intolerant to gluten. Research shows that, even in those without gluten intolerance, gluten becomes like "glue" in the digestive tract and can prevent nutrient absorption in the small intestine. Reducing the amount of gluten in the diet is a healthy idea for everyone. Grains without gluten are brown rice, teff, amaranth, buckwheat, millet, and one that is called a super grain, quinoa (actually a seed that is high in protein).

Eliminating white flour necessitates major changes in habits. As with sugar, the easy way to eliminate white flour is to eliminate processed foods. White flour is not a whole food, so if you switch to eating whole, unprocessed foods, you won't be consuming white flour. If forgoing white flour seems daunting, take it in stages. Decide which items to cut first—perhaps dinner rolls, biscuits, or bread. Gradually changing may encourage you to continue in a positive healthy direction. Drastic changes often result in a feeling of deprivation and lead to frustration, which is not conducive to long-term change.

Don't be fooled by phony "whole wheat" products. Most so-called whole-wheat products are not that at all. If you read the label carefully, you will find that this "healthy" product is really just white flour with a little whole wheat added along with some caramel coloring to make the white flour look darker.

A whole grain is a seed that can be sprouted or planted and will grow. A "whole grain" that cannot create life can no longer support life. That is why "whole-grain" breads and products at the store are not your best choice. Sprouted-grain products are better. Brown rice is a whole grain and is a healthful choice. White rice is a processed carbohydrate similar to white flour. The bran and germ, which contain most of the nutrients, have been stripped from white rice, making it another unfood. On the *NBFA* Lifestyle, choose organically grown brown rice, which is much more flavorful and satisfying, with the fiber and nutrients still intact, and it packs a chewy, nutty taste.

Tips to Help You Avoid Flour

- Don't buy processed breakfast cereals. Boxed breakfast cereals that are touted as healthy are still not good choices (even most of those found in a health-food store). Not only are they made with nutrient-deficient refined grains, but they contain added sugars and other toxic additives. Regardless of what you have been taught, they are not a healthy way to start your day. Check labels and be sure not to purchase any that contain artificial colors, synthetic vitamins, artificial flavors, preservatives, or hydrogenated oils—and almost all of them do. Absolutely never eat puffed grains: puffed wheat, puffed rice (including rice cakes), puffed amaranth, and puffed millet. The high temperature and pressure used to puff grain alters the molecular structure and makes it toxic. In his book *Fighting the Food Giants,* Paul Stitt reported an experiment in which rats were fed either whole wheat or puffed wheat. The rats eating the whole wheat lived more than a year while the rats eating the puffed wheat died within two weeks.

- Use whole grains in place of boxed cereals. Grains can be eaten without cooking by sprouting them or grinding and soaking them. They can be cooked whole in water, and topped with raw nuts or flaxseed, a little cinnamon, and stevia for sweetness. A milk alternative, such as fresh almond milk, tops it off. You can have great variety by experimenting with different grains, such as whole amaranth, quinoa, spelt, barley, buckwheat, oats, millet, brown rice, teff, and others. You may even try mixing a couple of grains. (See chapter 13 for cooking instructions.) Grains are not even necessary for breakfast. Fresh fruit along with raw nuts or seeds is a satisfying breakfast and also a time saver (real "fast food") on busy mornings.

- Replace white pastas with whole-grain pastas, or better, with whole grains. It is not difficult to find or adjust to whole-grain pastas. Many people like brown rice pasta better than whole wheat since it tastes more like "regular" pasta. Tinkyada is a brand that cooks well. (Read the label to be sure your pasta choice does not contain any form of white flour or white rice.) Once you have made this adjustment, try just a plain whole grain with your favorite pasta recipe. For example, make your pasta salad with organic brown rice, quinoa, bulgur wheat, barley, or millet in place of the pasta.

• Replace pasta with spaghetti squash or sautéed vegetables. Spaghetti squash can be baked (see chapter 13) and used in place of the pasta with a pesto, tomato, or garlic sauce. It is delicious and loaded with high-quality nutrition. With the low-carb craze, some Italian restaurants began offering their sauces on steamed vegetables rather than pasta. What a great idea to try at home!

• Since flour is often used as a thickening agent, it is hidden in many processed foods that you might not suspect. Always read labels and watch for hidden flour. Better yet, don't eat processed foods.

Good Things to Know About Bad Fats

Contrary to some popular dieting theories, fats and oils *are* a vital part of a healthy diet. Fats and oils are the primary materials used to form cell walls (membranes). Using the correct fats and oils, called essential fatty acids, to construct these membranes is fundamental to our biology. The correct ones have a special shape that allows them to fit together properly and perform their function in cell walls. They are essential for good health and mental function, while the wrong ones promote disease and weight gain. Even though most Americans eat a high-fat diet, we are deficient in healthy oils. As such, beware of diets that totally eliminate fats and oils. While deficient in healthy oils, we are overloaded with the wrong oils.

We eat excessive amounts of saturated animal fats and toxic processed oils along with processed foods containing these oils.

Most of the oils sold in supermarkets are processed oils; they are toxic and unhealthy. Supermarket oils usually contain excessive omega-6 oils and have been heated to high temperatures to bleach and deodorize them. Bleaching and deodorizing usually takes place at about 500 degrees, which makes the oils crystal clear and extends shelf life, but once you exceed 320 degrees, massive trans fat formation occurs. Above 392 degrees, powerful toxins called lipid peroxides are formed. There is no safe level of lipid peroxides or trans fats; both can severely damage cells.

Processing oils converts essential fatty acids into trans fats. Although similar in structure, the shape of trans fats is significantly different. When trans fats replace essential fatty acids in your cell walls, they interfere with normal cell functions. Picture trying to build a sturdy, leakproof brick wall with a heap of misshapen, irregular, and jagged bricks. Your body faces the same problem when it tries to form healthy cell membranes with trans fats in processed oils. Trans fats make these membranes leaky and brittle. As more and more cells in your body become leaky and brittle, you develop serious health problems. When essential fatty acids are not available and trans fats are, cells use what is available. The result is a defective cell wall that leaves the door wide open for malfunction and disease.

Almost all of the oils sold in supermarkets, and even most of those sold in health-food stores, are toxic and fail to provide your body what it needs. Trans fats are found in all kinds of commonly used oils: canola, corn, safflower, sunflower, soybean, and cottonseed. None of these oils are acceptable, and they are not part of the *NBFA* Lifestyle. All hydrogenated oils, including margarine and vegetable shortening, must be avoided for the same reasons. Again, read those labels, because these inappropriate oils are found in many foods.

The following is a list of foods almost guaranteed to contain unhealthy oils.

bakery items	hummus (most commercially
baking mixes	available varieties)
biscuit mixes	marinades
breads	mayonnaise
breakfast cereals	nutritional bars
chips of all varieties	peanut butter
chocolate and carob bars	pizzas
chocolate bars	toaster pastries
chocolate or carob chips	roasted nuts
coffee creamers	salad dressings
cookies (packaged)	sauces
crackers (most commercially	soups
available varieties)	tortillas (most commercially
French fries	available varieties)
guacamole (most commer-	yogurt (some)
cially available varieties)	yogurt raisins

This list could go on. Absolutely never choose any item with the words "hydrogenated" or "partially hydrogenated" on the label. Avoid sunflower, safflower, soybean, canola, cotton-seed, peanut, and corn oils; these oils are processed and also contain excessive omega-6s. Better yet, avoid all processed foods. Whole foods, such as avocado, coconut, olives, raw nuts, hemp seed, flaxseed, and other seeds have healthy oils. The more convenience foods you eat, the more processed oils you consume. A good rule of thumb is to avoid all fried foods, including French fries. Fast food and even upscale restaurant food is fried in poor-quality oil, high in trans fats and lipid peroxides.

When purchasing oil, don't be fooled by the words "cold pressed." This does not necessarily mean the oil is safe. Residues of toxic solvents, which are used to extract the oil, remain in the oil. Even oils that are not solvent extracted can be unhealthy. The friction resulting from the pressing process makes the oil become very hot, so that without adding heat the oil is still heated beyond what is safe. The heat generated in the extraction process oxidizes the oil, making it toxic. High-quality olive oil has not been heated or solvent extracted and is an excellent choice.

Omega-3 and Omega-6: A Balancing Act

By now, you may be asking where you could possibly find good fats and oils. For now, suffice it to say that the right oils include essential omega-3 and omega-6 fatty acids. Both omega-3 and omega-6 fatty acids are good for us, but only when consumed in the correct ratio. The Standard American Diet supplies far too much omega-6 and too little omega-3. This imbalanced ratio has an inflammatory effect, and inflammation is a common denominator in all chronic disease. Stop inflammation and you go a long way toward shutting off the disease process. Too many omega-6s initiate and perpetuate a disease-producing inflammatory process that contributes to overweight and aging.

Insufficient omega-3s can cause us to eat more sugar. A 2004 study in the *Journal of Nutritional Health and Aging* found that "a given level of perception of a sweet taste requires a larger quantity of sugar in subjects with alpha-linolenic acid [omega-3] deficiency." If you have a sweet tooth, you need more sugar to satisfy it if you are short on omega-3s.

Because of our enormous consumption of unhealthy oils, our ratio of omega-3s to 6s is way out of whack. Experts estimate that the proper ratio of 3s to 6s is ideally about 1 to 1. By 1935, the ratio in the average American diet had already increased to an unhealthy 1 to 8. Today, it is even more disastrous at 1 to 20, and for some people it is 1 to 50! This change in ratios is a major contributor to our disastrous increase in chronic disease. Research indicates that one out of five

Americans have so little omega-3s in their blood that it cannot even be measured by standard tests. The primary reason for this epidemic imbalance is our excessive consumption of the wrong oils—corn, sunflower, peanut, soy, canola, and safflower—largely in processed food. Chapter 4 lists foods with omega-3 fatty acids that you should include in your diet.

Another contributor to our imbalance of 3s and 6s is our increased consumption of make-believe fish, meat, and eggs. For example, most of the salmon available today has been farmed in an artificial environment where they are fed food with too much omega-6. Farmed fish do not eat the same diet as fish in their natural environment, which changes their chemistry. The same holds true for beef and chicken. Traditionally, cows have been fed on a diet of grass and hay, and chicken on insects, grass, and weeds. Today they are fed an unnatural diet of grains, which changes their natural fatty acid ratios. Consider that a real egg from a freely foraging chicken is a good source of DHA (an essential omega-3 fatty acid) and contains about 300 milligrams of DHA; the supermarket variety of make-believe eggs from grain-fed chickens averages only 18 milligrams. Nearly all cattle are shipped to feed lots prior to slaughter to feed them grains and fatten them up. If you eat this grain-finished beef, as most Americans do, you will be getting too much omega-6. Fortunately, there is a growing demand for grass-fed, grass-finished beef, which has made it economically feasible for more ranchers to return to older and healthier methods of animal husbandry.

The Trouble with Dairy and Excess Animal Protein

The last of the Big Four are dairy products and excess animal protein, which are considered together. Both dairy and other animal protein have led most of us down an unhealthy path, and those who consume dairy products or eat animal protein more than a couple of times a week are much more likely to gain weight. Even worse, excess animal protein promotes cancer. Americans have been terribly misled into consuming far too much animal protein; this includes meat, dairy, eggs, and fish. We have also seen weight-loss diets that make animal protein the hero and carbohydrates the villain. The negative effects of these tragic errors have been catastrophic, contributing to our epidemic of cancer, overweight, heart disease, diabetes, and other chronic diseases.

Animal protein contributes to overweight disease by altering the way the body handles calories. Diets that are high in animal protein and fat (the typical American diet) cause the body to store more calories as fat, while low-protein diets trigger our bodies to burn more calories. Animal protein also causes an increase in insulin, resulting in an exaggerated insulin response to carbohydrates when consumed along with the protein in the meal—one reason that eating meat with potatoes is a bad idea. Animal protein also has an acidic effect on cellular pH.

Animal protein is not all bad. The science indicates it can be safely and beneficially consumed in small quantities. A good rule is to use animal protein as a condiment, not as a main course. You do not need to consume animal protein at every meal or even every day. Rather, you should get most of your protein from plant-based foods. Most people have been so conditioned to think of meat and dairy as their source of protein that they don't realize there is high-quality, easily absorbable protein in plant foods. Consider this: A 100-calorie portion of vegetables such as broccoli, spinach, and kale has more protein than 100 calories of sirloin steak. Vegetables, beans, lentils, and grains are all good sources of protein.

Minimizing animal protein is essential for maintaining health and normal weight. The average American consumes about 15 percent of his or her calories as protein, with about

80 percent of that from animal sources. By contrast, healthier populations in rural China get less than 10 percent of their calories from protein, and only 10 percent of that is from animal sources. This huge difference in the amount of animal protein consumed has profound health consequences.

The Recommended Daily Allowance (RDA) for total protein is 50 to 60 grams per day. For safety purposes in allowing for unique individual needs, the RDA is a little more than twice our actual need. Most of us can get along just fine with half the RDA. However, many Americans get twice the RDA, and our average consumption of animal protein alone is about 70 grams per day. Think about it, Americans average more animal protein than the RDA for total protein. By contrast, most rural Chinese, who are far healthier than we, average 7 grams of animal protein per day or ten times less. What is the effect of excess animal protein? Cancer, obesity, heart disease, diabetes, osteoporosis, and kidney, eye, brain, and autoimmune diseases. Given these problems, averaging 7 grams or less per day of animal protein appears a worthy goal. The remainder of our protein consumption should be plant protein, the primary sources of which are beans, peas, lentils, unrefined grains, seeds, nuts, and green vegetables.

The largest and most comprehensive nutrition study ever conducted is the China Study. World-renowned nutrition researcher T. Colin Campbell wrote a book with this title to bring that groundbreaking research to the public. Though Dr. Campbell grew up on a dairy farm believing that a diet rich in animal products was healthy, his research was so provoking that he became a vegan (someone who eats no animal products at all). Here are some of Dr. Campbell's conclusions:

- Animal protein, in excess of the amount needed for growth, promotes cancer.
- Low-animal-protein diets inhibit cancer formation and dramatically block cancer growth.

- People who eat the most animal-based foods suffer the most chronic disease.
- Even relatively small intakes of animal-based food are associated with adverse effects.
- Cow's milk protein (casein) is an exceptionally potent cancer promoter.
- A diet high in animal-based foods raises the risk of Alzheimer's disease.
- There are virtually no nutrients in animal-based foods that are not better provided by plants.

Make-Believe Meats

If consuming excess animal protein isn't bad enough, the meat and animal products currently offered at most stores are not even real meat, but rather make-believe meat. It may look like meat, but it does not contain the correct nutrients because it is commercially farmed. Current farming techniques focus on big business and large profits. Commercially farmed chickens, cows, and pigs are raised and fed in deplorable conditions. Many of these ill-treated animals never see real sunlight but live in a facility where they are so crowded with other animals that they are hardly able to move, much less exercise. They are pumped full of antibiotics and other drugs to keep them alive in their abusive, contaminated environment. They receive toxic feed consisting of animal by-products and recycled waste and are pumped full of hormones to stimulate rapid growth. These animals are fed large quantities of feed loaded with pesticides and other dangerous chemicals, which concentrate in the animals and poison us when we eat them. All this is done so agribusiness can profit from lower feed costs and accelerated time to slaughter. Even fish are now being farmed in containments that restrict movement and are given growth hormones to speed processing. Under these conditions, 90 percent of chickens have cancer when slaughtered, 80 percent of pigs have pneumonia, and a large percentage of cattle also have cancer. How could we possibly think that eating meat, fish, and eggs from diseased animals is healthy?

Farmed salmon is deficient in omega-3 fatty acids and high in PCBs and other contaminants. This type of farming is now being recognized as a significant environmental hazard. A study reported in the January 2005 issue of *Science* found that farmed salmon contained substantially more toxins than salmon caught in the wild. Shockingly, most of the "wild" salmon on the market is actually farmed. Avoid salmon unless you are confident of the source.

Processing plants—which manufacture lunchmeats, hot dogs, sausage, pepperoni, smoked meats, and bacon—add sugar, salt, and preservatives such as nitrates and nitrites to the already unhealthy meat. Nitrates and nitrites, when combined with stomach acid, can be transformed into potent carcinogens called nitrosamines. These additives damage the brain and the liver. You should absolutely avoid processed meats with nitrates and nitrites.

The average person consumes 80 to 90 percent of their pesticide residues from animal products, including meat, dairy, and eggs. Animal products are huge contributors to our ever-increasing toxic load due to the pesticides on the food that is fed to the animals, as well as to the hormones and drugs they are given. Toxins impair the body's attempts to find its correct weight.

How to Cut Down on Animal Protein

- Begin to introduce more vegan meals, which contain no animal products. (See chapter 13 for ideas.)
- Build meals around fresh, raw healthy salads as the main course, rather than meats. A small amount of high-quality animal protein or protein-rich sprouts can be added to your main-course salad.
- Avocados contain good essential fats and can be used to replace meat in meals.

- Nuts and seeds (raw and soaked/sprouted) are a good source of protein and healthy fat, which can be satisfying.
- Lentils easily replace ground beef in Mexican recipes, shepherd's pies, meatballs, and stuffed peppers. (See chapter 13.)
- If you do eat meat, make sure it is not grilled, charred, or browned in any way. Barbecuing meat is the most toxic way to prepare it. When fat drips into an open flame, dangerous cancer-causing chemicals called polycyclic aromatic hydrocarbons are formed. All proteins cooked at high temperatures contain several chemicals that have been proven to cause cancer in laboratory animals. Meat that is cooked at high temperatures produces carcinogens called heterocyclic aromatic amines.
- When you cook meat it is best to slow cook it at a low temperature for several hours. Using a crockpot and cooking on low for many hours or overnight is well-suited to this lifestyle.

Got Milk? Get Rid of It!

Most Americans have been brainwashed when it comes to dairy products. We grew up believing that milk, cheese, and yogurt were vital to health. The first time someone suggested that dairy products were not healthy, we thought they were crazy. In reality, modern milk is a highly toxic and allergenic make-believe food. The milk available in our stores contains undesirable hormones, antibiotics, pesticides, herbicides, PCBs, dioxins, viruses, and excessive bacteria, not to mention animal protein, including cancer-promoting casein. No one should be drinking this dangerous beverage or eating products made from milk.

Mothers are often advised to feed their children a quart of milk per day. Unfortunately, millions of us have paid a high price for this misguided advice. Television commercials tell us that milk "does a body good." News stories tell us to drink milk to ensure proper calcium intake. Recent commercials seek to convince dieters that milk and dairy products will help them lose weight. Think about that one. How could a food that was specifically designed to cause a calf to grow from ninety pounds to two thousand pounds in two years make you lose weight? Talk about misinformation! The truth is the opposite: milk makes you fat.

Dairy products are not included in the *NBFA* Lifestyle. Entire books have been devoted to teaching readers that milk does not do a body good (see *Don't Drink Your Milk* by pediatrician Frank Oski).

Remember when we talked about eating sugar and the negative effects of insulin on your body, including promoting cancer? Milk also increases insulin levels. Milk promotes type 2 diabetes, and milk drinkers suffer higher rates of diabetes and metabolic syndrome. Milk and dairy products sabotage your efforts to lose weight and maintain a healthy weight.

Where Will I Get My Calcium?

If you quit eating dairy products, you may wonder where you will get your calcium. We ask you this, "Where does a cow get her calcium?" From grass, right? The cow, whose milk is so rich in calcium, does not consume milk. Where does the 70 percent of the world's population that does not drink milk get their calcium? They get it from vegetables. Green vegetables, such as kale, broccoli, and collard greens, are loaded with calcium. Joel Fuhrman, M.D., writes in *Eat to Live,* "Many green vegetables have calcium-absorption rates of over 50 percent, compared with about 32 percent for milk. Additionally, since animal protein induces calcium excretion in the urine, calcium from milk is lost while the calcium retention from vegetables is higher. All green vegetables are high in calcium."

Helpful Suggestions for Discarding Dairy Products

- Use healthy milk substitutes in recipes, on whole grain cereals, or in any way you formerly used cow's or goat's milk. Almond milk, cashew milk, sesame seed milk, buckwheat milk, and brown rice milk are options that can be quickly and easily made in a blender. Beware of processed milk substitutes available in stores, as most of them have unhealthy preservatives or unnecessary sweeteners, and most are made with water containing toxic fluoride.
- If you want a drink that will give you a real boost in absorbable calcium and protein, try freshly made vegetable juices, especially green juices. Many health- food stores have a juice bar where you can purchase green juice that is made to order, or you can get your own juicer and juice your own organic veggie juice. This is optimal cell food!
- If you are an ice cream lover, do not despair. You can make delicious ice cream, milk shakes, and frozen treats from very ripe, frozen bananas.
- Try cheeseless veggie pizzas made on whole-grain crust. Top the pizza with a smorgasbord of favorite vegetable combinations including fresh tomatoes, mushrooms, bell peppers, banana peppers, onions, fresh garlic, zucchini, eggplant, spinach, artichokes, even broccoli.
- Delicious vegetable dip creations may be made without sour cream, cream, or other dairy products.

Recipes for the above appear in chapter 13.

Caffeine

Though it is not an official member of the Big Four, caffeine deserves mention for being a highly addictive, health-ravaging toxin. Caffeine, found in coffee, tea, soft drinks, chocolate, and other foods, is the most popular drug in the Western world. Soft drinks are a major source of caffeine. Caffeine is a component of many diet pills and is also added to many over-the-counter drugs such as allergy, cold, headache, and stay-awake preparations. Coffee is a particularly bad source of caffeine. Coffee contains a constellation of toxic chemicals that are known to disrupt the central nervous, cardiovascular, and respiratory systems, along with causing irritability and mood swings and being associated with liver cancer. One cup of coffee per day can usually be tolerated by most people, but drinking several cups of coffee or cola drinks is almost certain to cause harm. In pregnant women, just one cup of coffee per day is known to increase the risk of birth defects, low birth weight, premature delivery, and spontaneous abortion.

Caffeine is a stimulant from the same family as nicotine and morphine. As a stimulant, it increases heart rate and sometimes triggers irregular heartbeats, and leads to high blood pressure and increased insulin production. As caffeine revs up the system, false energy is supplied, but it also stimulates and increases appetite. With chronic caffeine use, the amount needed to achieve the effect increases.

Caffeine also sabotages weight loss by depleting nutrients, including the B vitamins (needed for stress), calcium (needed for bones), and iron (needed to prevent anemia), as well as magnesium, potassium, and zinc. The resulting nutrient deficiency increases appetite. Caffeine reduces hydrochloric acid in the stomach, contributing to a number of digestive disorders as well.

Most people don't need to be convinced that caffeine is bad for them, but the addiction is powerful and cannot be broken overnight. As you prepare for the *NBFA* Lifestyle, you will find a section in chapter 12 to help you wean yourself off of caffeine. It needs to be a gradual withdrawal, and products like Teeccino (an acceptable coffee substitute) can be extremely helpful.

The Fast-Food Track to Overweight

Do fast foods make you fat? Numerous studies and common sense say they do. Fast foods are rich in calories, and excess calories make you fat. Morgan Spurlock's 2004 documentary *Super Size Me* showed just how dramatic this effect can be. In one month of eating exclusively at McDonald's, Spurlock gained more than twenty-five pounds, developed a medically alarming fatty liver condition, increased his cholesterol, and lost his libido. If you have not viewed this movie, we encourage you to do so.

Feeling satisfied depends on the size of a meal rather than the calories it contains. Fast food confuses the body's appetite control mechanism because the calories are concentrated in less bulk. A similar size fast-food meal can have at least twice the calories of a home-prepared meal. When you eat fiber-deficient fast food, by the time you feel full you have consumed far too many calories. Consider that a McDonald's meal consisting of a Big Mac (590 calories), large fries (540 calories), a large cola (310 calories), and a caramel sundae for dessert (360 calories), adds up to 1,800 calories at one meal. Contrast this to one-third pound of halibut (188 calories), a quarter pound of broccoli (28 calories), a quarter pound of salad (20 calories), oil and vinegar dressing (50 calories), and an apple for dessert (53 calories). *This nutritious, appetite-satisfying meal adds up to only 339 calories.* This is 1,461 calories less than the McDonald's meal and 721 calories less than a Double Whopper at Burger King. Meanwhile, the healthy meal supplies a vast improvement in nutrition, all without the health-damaging toxins contained in fast food. As you can see, real food gives you more nutrients, fewer calories, and fewer toxins, keeping you healthier and thinner.

A six-year study, reported in the January 1, 2005, issue of the medical journal *Lancet,* found that study participants who consumed fast food twice a week or more gained more weight and exhibited twice the increase in insulin resistance compared to those who ate fast food less than once a week. Fast food makes you gain weight and increases your risk of developing insulin resistance and type 2 diabetes.

Here's to Good Health and Great Taste

Changing your diet in order to eat for good health and long life—and weight loss—is not that difficult, especially if you make changes step by step. You will find new food choices that are filling and delicious. A better understanding of the devastating consequences inside your body caused by the foods that you used to love and thought were fairly healthy may give you incentive. The two most important choices to make: *do not* eat processed foods, and *do* eat large quantities of nutrient-rich plant foods, including fruits, vegetables, grains, beans, seeds, and nuts. This approach helps you get off the Big Four, reduce sodium intake, and alkalize and supply your cells with the nutrients they need to achieve permanent weight control and wellness.

FOODS THAT ENERGIZE, REPAIR, AND KEEP YOU TRIM

Now it's time to learn more about the variety of wholesome foods that you are encouraged to eat, where to find them, and how to prepare them. These are the best "diet secrets" for successful and healthy weight loss:

- Eat for color: green, red, orange, purple, and white.
- Fiber is critical, and you should know how to get plenty of it.
- Organic food is necessary, and certain foods are most important to find organic.
- Raw/living vegetables, fruits, nuts, and seeds are foundational to any healthy lifestyle; incorporate them into your meals.
- Essential fatty acids are crucial to weight loss.

- How you eat is important too—from what is eaten first, to how you chew, and when and what you drink.
- Water is vital to life and weight loss.

Man does not die—he commits slow suicide with his unnatural habits of living. Your body is the most gloriously accurate instrument of this universe. Given the correct fuel, pure air, exercise, and keeping it internally clean, your body will last indefinitely and function perfectly.

—Paul Bragg

After reading the previous chapters and realizing how many foods make you fat and sick, you are likely asking, "What is left to eat?" The answer is plenty—plenty of "real" food. And if you have found yourself bored with your choices on other "diets," lost in your search for interesting meals, and hungry most of the time, don't despair. Super foods to the rescue!

Meals can still be satisfying and delicious. At first, you will need to adjust because processed food corrupts taste buds with its abundance of salt, sugar, and other additives such as MSG. Once your system resets itself, you will learn to appreciate and enjoy whole foods in a brand-new way. Sweet red bell peppers can be a crispy, crunchy, and sweet indulgence. A ripe, juicy mango can be savored as an incredibly appealing treat. Raw nuts and seeds will soon be a greatly anticipated snack food. Not only will whole foods take on a new image, you will also learn to fix pleasurable meals with whole foods. It does not happen overnight, but you will be given a head start with the recipes offered in chapter 13.

Nature provides a wide array of foods that are full of powerful antioxidants, phytochemicals, minerals, vitamins, and enzymes that reduce the risk of disease, slow aging, invigorate your body, and help you stay trim. Life goes on—in fact, much higher quality life—without the destructive Big Four and processed junk food. The key words to remember: *fresh, whole, unprocessed, raw, organic, vegetables, fruits, grains,* and *legumes.*

Overweight individuals often cut down on the amount of food they eat without changing the types of foods they eat. That is a recipe for failure. Calorie reduction without nutrient addition is counterproductive because that approach typically increases malnourishment (deficiency) and encourages food cravings. If you want to lose weight and maintain a healthy weight, you must consume foods with a high amount of nutrition per calorie. *Make your calories count rather than counting calories.*

Looking for Nutrients? Look for Color

The *NBFA* Lifestyle is, for the most part, a plant-based, whole-foods way of eating. Plant-based whole foods are foods as we find them in nature, and they are perfectly suited to meet our biological needs. This is the food that nature intended to make up the bulk of our intake. If you cannot always eat fresh, raw, whole foods, be sure to make choices that keep your food in its closest state to nature. Our bodies were not designed to thrive on processed food, which has become commonplace in the last century along with our epidemic of chronic disease and overweight. In his book, *Eat to Live,* Dr. Joel Fuhrman states, "The greater the quantity and assortment of fruits and vegetables consumed, the lower the incidence of heart attacks, strokes and cancer. . . . There is one thing we know for sure: raw vegetables and fresh fruits have powerful anti-cancer agents."

One compelling reason for a plant-based diet is the necessity of phytochemicals—plant chemicals derived from the pigments in plants. The most brightly colored fruits and vegetables contain the most phytochemicals and provide the most health benefit. Some phytochemicals that you have probably heard of are lycopene, found in tomatoes, and carotene, found in carrots and other yellow/orange vegetables. Research is revealing that phytochemicals provide protection from diseases such as cancer, heart disease, diabetes, Alzheimer's, and more. More than one thousand phytochemicals have been discovered, and new ones are being found all the time. A single serving of a vegetable or fruit contains many such nutrients. An orange, for example, not only provides the antioxidant vitamin C, but also has more than 170 phytochemicals along with potassium, thiamine, and folate. A carrot contains more than 217 phytochemicals, a tomato more than 300, and an apple more than 150.

Obtaining a variety of phytochemicals is important because they play many critical roles in the body. Numerous phytochemicals are among the over fifteen hundred known antioxidants that provide cellular protection by neutralizing free radicals that would otherwise damage our genes and tissues and weaken our ability to self-repair. Other useful phytochemicals include isoflavones, which function like hormones. Indoles (found in cabbage) stimulate enzymes. Saponins (found in legumes) inhibit the multiplication of cancer cells, and allicin (found in garlic) has antibacterial properties. This illustrates the importance of consuming a wide array of vegetables and fruits to obtain the greatest number of phytochemicals possible, and also to take advantage of the synergy as they act in combination.

While each phytochemical provides unique benefits, they are even more powerful when they work in combination. Evidence is now overwhelming that common vitamins, minerals, and plant chemicals interfere with the cancer process at every level. Many chemicals found in plant foods are capable of turning cancer cells back into normal cells. Certain flavonoids found in vegetables have been found to suppress and even to kill cancer cells. In fact, food and nutritional supplements have a far more powerful effect on cancer than chemotherapy. Be sure to eat vegetables and fruits from all of the basic color groups: green (the darker the better—consider spinach, kale, collard greens, broccoli, cabbage, asparagus, watercress, Swiss chard, Brussels sprouts, and bok choy), blue/purple (eggplant, plums, blueberries, blackberries, and grapes), red (beets, bell peppers, tomatoes, cranberries, raspberries, watermelon, and strawberries), orange/yellow (carrots, sweet potatoes, pumpkin, winter squash, mangos, papaya, and oranges), and white (onions, garlic, turnip, jicama, and cauliflower).

Growing your own vegetables and fruit, or visiting a farmer's market are the best options. Most local farmers harvest produce hours before selling it at a green market, as opposed to days, weeks, or even years for food in a supermarket. If you must rely on a health store, find out what day the produce arrives so that you can acquire it when it is as fresh as possible. When fresh is not available, frozen is the next, but less nutritious, option. We recommend you avoid anything in cans because it has minimal nutrition and more toxins. Want fast food? Consider an apple. What could be quicker than biting into a fresh, crispy apple, a baby carrot, or a juicy cucumber? No drive-thru, no cooking, no can opener, no dicing, grating, or blending. Eating these foods without peeling (when organic) increases the fiber and nutrient content.

Fiber Staves Off Hunger—And Disease

A vital component of plants is fiber. Only plant foods contain fiber; there is no fiber in animal products. Fiber is the indigestible part of plants that has no calories and cannot be absorbed by the cells, yet it is crucial to the healthy functioning of the digestive system because it provides bulk. Bulk makes you feel full and shuts off the appetite while assisting in absorption and keeping things moving through your digestive system. These functions are keys to successful weight management. There are two types of fiber: soluble and insoluble.

Soluble fiber—including pectin, gums, and hemicelluloses—attracts water, which slows digestion to a rate at which nutrients can be efficiently absorbed from the stomach and intestine. This type of fiber is found in plants such as nuts, seeds, beans, lentils, peas, barley, and some fruits and vegetables. Soluble fiber helps slow the absorption of sugar from the gut, thereby preventing insulin spikes, which make you store fat. Soluble fiber is fermented by bacteria in the large intestine, helping to support healthy flora in the gut, as well as helping them to produce beneficial B-complex vitamins. This fermentation also produces short-chain fatty acids that are required to keep gut cells healthy.

The other type of fiber is insoluble. Consisting of polysaccharides found in most whole grains and vegetables, insoluble fiber speeds the movement of waste, adds bulk, and prevents constipation.

Most Americans do not consume enough fiber. When the bulk of your calories comes from refined foods and animal products, fiber is lacking, and constipation (whether realized or not) is prevalent. Fiber is essential to health since so much disease begins with an unhealthy colon, everything from the obvious—colitis, diverticulitis, and colon cancers—to the not-so-obvious—headaches, seizures, heart disease, and brain cancers. Many people have unhealthy colons that harbor pounds of backed-up, putrefying waste. It is critical to flush out old waste and acquire the fiber needed to keep the bowels moving while also contributing to the feeling of fullness. When plant fiber figures prominently in your daily diet, you become healthier and lose weight.

Organic: Tipping the Scales in Your Favor

There are three main reasons that organic foods are the better bargain for your health: they contain more nutrients and fewer toxins, and they taste better. Organic foods contain more nutrients, including minerals such as iron, potassium, and magnesium. Continuous cropping and the use of artificial fertilizers have resulted in American farm soils being the worst in the world for mineral content; we are growing food that often lacks some of the basic minerals needed to sustain life. Organic farming helps to restore minerals to the soil, resulting in plants having more minerals, vitamins, antioxidants, phytochemicals, and other nutrients. In the Organic Center's January 2005 *State of Science Review,* Charles Benbrook, the center's chief scientist, concluded that, on average, antioxidant levels are 30 percent higher in organic food compared to conventional food grown under similar conditions. Several studies discovered that levels of specific vitamins, flavonoids, or antioxidants in organic foods were two to three times that in conventional products. You can increase your antioxidant and nutrient intake simply by switching to organic.

Organic foods contain fewer toxins. Consider the trauma you introduce to your cells when you ingest foods that are full of chemicals, herbicides, pesticides, fungicides, growth hormones, and so on. This is especially important to children because their small bodies are more susceptible to toxins than adult bodies. Because pesticides are neurotoxic, they can damage developing nervous systems. As we were writing this chapter, preliminary results were released from one of the first studies to measure the effect of pesticides on children's brains. This study, sponsored by the National Institutes of Health and conducted by the University of North Dakota, found that children who live on farms, or within one mile of a farm, performed significantly lower on IQ tests than their peers. These children also had lower scores on verbal comprehension, visual perceptual reasoning, memory, and mental processing speed. We are feeding our children food that is contaminated with pesticides, and then we wonder why they are not doing well in school, cannot compete in science and mathematics internationally, and why they are fat. (More on pesticides and overweight in chapter 6.)

A 2005 study reported in *Environmental Health Perspectives* measured the effects of organic food on the pesticide levels in schoolchildren. Children ate their normal diets and were then measured for pesticide levels in their blood. Next the children were fed organic foods for five days and were measured again. The pesticide levels dropped to negligible levels in just five days. One child went from 263 ppb of Malathion to 1.6 ppb. "In conclusion," the researchers said, "we were able to demonstrate that an organic diet provides a dramatic and immediate protective effect against exposure to organophosphate pesticides." A USDA study in 1990 found that 75 percent of conventionally grown food contained pesticide residues, while only 23 percent of organic foods measured positive. Whenever you eat conventional foods, your body must go on the offensive, using up precious nutrients that are already in short supply in order to protect you from the toxins. If you must eat conventionally produced food, at least wash it well and peel when able.

Although conventional plant foods are contaminated with toxins, the majority of consumers incorrectly believe that chemically treated vegetables and fruits pose the biggest threat in their diets. However, an estimated 80 percent of the toxic pesticides and chemicals in American diets come from animal products (meat and dairy), not plant foods. When you think of organic, you must consider not only plant foods, but animal products.

Organic food tastes better. Consumers usually report organic food is richer in flavor. This flavor is not always noticed when first switching to organic, but more so when consuming a conventional fruit or vegetable after one has grown accustomed to eating organic. Many animals are smarter than humans when it comes to organic food; they prefer it and choose it when given the option. In a 2003 study conducted at the Copenhagen Zoo and published in the journal *Oekologisk Jordbrug* (*Organic Agriculture*), zookeeper Niels Melchiorsen reported that monkeys and chimpanzees are able to tell the difference between organic and conventional produce. "Their choice is not at all random," he said. "The chimpanzees are able to tell the difference between the organic and regular fruit. If we give them organic and traditional bananas, they systematically choose the organic bananas, which they eat with the skin on. But they peel the traditional bananas before eating them." There have been numerous published scientific feeding trials done with rats, rabbits, and chickens that consistently show the same results.

We all know that organic products cost more money, but consider this: you have to consume, on average, two or three pieces of conventional fruit or servings of conventional vegetables to get the same amount of nutrition in one serving of organic. Since you are eating to get nutrition, eating organic is the better bargain. Then consider the calories. If an average orange has 80 calories and you choose to consume conventional oranges, not only do you bring toxic enemies into your body, but you must consume two or three of the oranges, meaning double or triple the calories, to get the antioxidants you could have acquired, without toxins, in one organic orange with 80 calories. Since most people are not going to consume two to three times the amount of food, the result is nutritional deficiency and disease. In truth, if you cut processed foods out of your diet, the savings will be so great that organic foods become affordable. Cutting out milk, sodas, bread, cookies, chips, ice cream, and other toxic processed foods and excess animal protein will save you so much that people often find that they are not only eating better, but they have cut their food costs. Consider what a package of toxic breakfast cereal costs per pound versus organic whole grains, and you will quickly see how big your savings can be.

Seek out organic foods in your area and online. Eat as many of your foods organic as possible. *Animal products should not be consumed if they cannot be obtained from an organic source.* So many brands of meat, poultry, and fish proclaim they are free-range or hormone- and antibiotic-free. Such a claim is not enough. Most free-range, hormone-free animals are fed toxic, chemical-laden feeds, rather than being raised naturally, grazing on untreated grassland. Certified organic products come from animals that have not been fed chemically treated grains. Check out smaller farms and health stores in your region.

Many farmer's markets feature some farmers who grow organically. At a farmer's market, you can at least ask how the produce is grown and when it was harvested. The nutrient quality of food deteriorates with each passing hour after harvest. The closer to harvest that you can consume produce, the more nutrients you will find in the food. By the time it goes through the distribution system and reaches a supermarket, its nutritional value has been substantially diminished, sometimes even eliminated. Buying straight from the farmer also gives you a better chance of getting produce that was picked ripe rather than harvested prematurely to survive the distribution process. When it comes to produce, you may not find all varieties organic. At times you may choose for variety, even if it is not all organic. Following is a list of crops that are usually sprayed more heavily and products that usually require fewer chemicals. Use this as a guide for conventional items that are safer to substitute when their organic counterparts are not available. Certain heavily sprayed crops, such as strawberries, should be avoided if you cannot find them organic, fresh, and local (fresh berries are essential since berries mold rapidly).

Heavily Treated Fruits
apples
apricots
cherries
dates
grapes
hot peppers
lemons
nectarines
peaches
pears
raspberries
strawberries

Heavily Treated Vegetables
bell peppers
cabbage
carrots
celery
cucumbers
green beans
potatoes
spinach
sweet potatoes

Less-Treated Fruits
bananas
blueberries
figs
grapefruit
kiwi fruit
mangoes
papayas
pineapples
plantains
plums
watermelons

Less-Treated Vegetables
asparagus
avocados
broccoli
brussels sprouts
cauliflower
eggplant
garlic
okra
onions
radishes

Find Out How Your Meat and Fish Were Raised

As we've said, when it comes to buying meat, poultry, and fish, we advise you to choose organic or to skip meat and fish entirely. Because most of the pesticide residues we ingest are from animal products, this is an area where there is not room for compromise if you want to be healthy and maintain normal weight. Not only do beef, pork, and poultry contain pesticides, hormones, and disease-causing parasites, but fish, so often touted as healthy, has significant problems, especially farmed fish.

Fish is usually considered to be a healthy food, but in 2004 several studies questioned the safety of farmed salmon. In January 2005, a study in the prestigious academic journal *Science* found that farmed salmon contained ten times the amount of suspected carcinogens as wild salmon, including polychlorinated biphenyls (PCBs), pesticides, flame retardants, and dioxins. These toxins come from the contaminated food fed to the captive fish, which also includes antibiotics, artificial dyes, and hormones. These toxins are known to bioaccumulate in your fatty tissues, along with all the other fat-soluble toxins you are accumulating, which over time reach dangerous concentrations. Such toxins can interfere with weight control. In addition, pregnant women or nursing mothers will pass these toxins on to their children. Such toxins are especially dangerous to children, causing a variety of consequences including cancer, immune suppression, lower IQs, and learning and behavioral problems. A study commissioned by the Environmental Working Group found that farmed salmon was contaminated with PCBs an average of sixteen times higher than wild salmon and four times the amount found in beef, making it the most PCB-contaminated protein source.

But if you think you are eating wild salmon, look closely. As it turns out, much of the "wild" salmon on the market is actually farmed. In April 2005, the *New York Times* published an exposé based on tests it had commissioned. Investigators purchased "wild" salmon from New York City stores at an average price of nineteen dollars per pound. The fish was sent to a laboratory for analysis. Seventy-five percent of that expensive "wild" salmon was actually farmed. Farmed salmon now constitutes 90 percent of salmon sales in the United States. Avoid eating any farmed fish, and be especially vigilant to determine the true source of your "wild" salmon.

Raw Foods Are Teeming with Life

Raw plant food is often referred to as living food because it contains biologically active components, such as enzymes, phytochemicals, and hormones. When eaten raw, optimal nutrition is preserved. Once you begin to alter food by chopping or heating, its living components begin to disappear. Living foods energize you, while cooking deactivates critical nutrients. The food may look essentially the same, but nutrients are fragile and easily lost or devalued. Our foods are already so nutrient-deficient that cooking them makes a bad situation even worse. Proteins, phytonutrients, vitamins, minerals, fats, and carbohydrates are all degraded by heat, and at times even become toxic. Typically 30 to 40 percent of the minerals are lost, as well as 20 to 50 percent of the vitamins. Most sensitive to this destructive process are vitamins, co-enzymes, and enzymes.

All life, both plant and animal, is dependent upon enzymes. Enzymes enable your body to produce energy for all of its functions, from digestion to the removal of toxins, to activities as simple as blinking an eye or breathing. You cannot move a finger or sustain a thought without enzymes. Biologically active enzymes are only acquired through uncooked foods because enzymes are very heat sensitive. Food enzymes start to deactivate at 105 degrees Fahrenheit and are completely deactivated at 130 degrees. The temperature of steam is 212 degrees, and cooking temperatures usually exceed 300 degrees. Therefore, all living, revitalizing enzymes are destroyed in cooking. Cooking also alters other nutrients, making many of them biologically unavailable to our bodies. Worse still, enzymes are essential for the digestion and utilization of all other nutrients. Eating cooked food stresses the body, forcing it to manufacture extra enzymes in order to digest it and to compensate for the enzymes lost in the cooking process. Only fifty years ago our society ate a much larger percentage of raw, unprocessed food than we do today. As we have decreased consumption of raw fruits and vegetables and accelerated the use of processed foods, overweight and disease have increased.

Cooked food actually suppresses the immune system. After eating cooked food, the blood immediately shows an increase in white blood cells, which are our body's first line of defense. Cooked food appears to be so alien that it provokes an immune response. Scientist Udo Erasmus, author of *Fats and Oils*, wrote:

> When cooked (or dead) food is eaten, a defense reaction occurs in the tissues of the stomach and digestive tract. This reaction is similar to the reaction we find in infections and around tumors and involves the accumulation of white blood cells, swelling, and fever-like increase in temperature of the stomach and intestinal tissues. [As a result, we] experience tiredness after the meal. The same reaction takes place when half the food is eaten raw, but the cooked part is eaten first. When the raw part of the food is eaten first, however, this reaction does not take place.

Therefore, when we eat a meal, the raw food should be consumed first in order to prevent such an immune response. Always begin each meal with some sort of salad or raw vegetable entrée.

Raw food satisfies nutritional needs, which helps to control your appetite and maintain healthy weight. Certain cooking methods are particularly detrimental to your health. Browning and blackening foods causes them to form powerful carcinogens. Microwaving changes the molecular composition of foods, decreasing nutrients and creating toxins. The energy of the microwaves breaks apart the water molecules within the food, causing them to react with the food in ways they would not otherwise do. Some of the unnatural molecules created are toxic. When you do cook food, it is best to use low temperatures and longer cooking times. Steaming and slow cookers are suited for this purpose. Dehydrators can slightly heat foods to temperatures below 108 degrees, preserving nutrients and enzymes, yet still warming food.

Your goal should be to continually increase your consumption of raw vegetables, fruits, nuts, seeds, and grains. Most people do not even eat as many fresh fruits and vegetables as the food pyramid recommends, and that recommendation falls woefully short of what is needed. Dr. Russell Blaylock, in his book *Natural Strategies for Cancer Patients,* writes: "In terms of health benefits, eating fewer than five servings of fruits and vegetables a day does very little good. The health benefits begin at five servings, and, for people below the age of fifty, they reach a maximum at ten servings. For those over the age of fifty, adding two additional servings—that is, consuming a total of twelve servings a day—provides the maximum health benefits." Sadly, average Americans eat only about 5 percent of food as raw fruits and vegetables, when they really need a minimum of 75 percent. The tomato or lettuce on a cheeseburger is all of the raw food some consume in an entire day. What's worse, ketchup is the only "vegetable" some individuals eat in an entire day. Some people go for days on end with no raw, living food and very few cooked vegetables. No wonder we face a health crisis in our country.

Don't Create a Digestive Traffic Jam

Since raw food contains enzymes necessary for its digestion, it does not tax our system the way cooked food does. It moves much more rapidly through the digestive tract. Raw organic foods also are free from the toxins and preservatives that processed foods introduce. It takes hard work and precious enzymes to move dead, cooked, and processed foods through the digestive tract. Some cooked foods can take forty to one hundred hours to move through your system. The energy saved when raw food is eaten can be used for other bodily functions, such as healing or providing vigor for daily tasks. This helps to explain why you feel tired or drowsy after eating a big meal of cooked foods. The digestion of that meal consumes your energy. Increased energy will encourage you to exercise more and to stay committed to your new way of eating. Notice how much lighter, more energetic, and sharp-minded you feel after eating a meal of all raw foods.

Consider the story of Heather, who worked for a catering business. She was seeking to implement the *NBFA* Lifestyle by eliminating the Big Four and consuming more living food. At times, this was not easy for her since the servers at catered events were permitted to eat for free after serving and before cleaning up. As tempting as the free and readily available food was, Heather made an encouraging observation. She would take a large salad and other raw foods to eat while the other employees ate the catered food. After eating, none of them had much energy to clean up, but she still felt great.

More Whole Grains, Less Unwanted Fat

Studies have shown that diets rich in whole grains and dietary fiber may be a key component in reducing and preventing obesity. According to a 2001 Louisiana State University study, the amount of fiber in the diet is the greatest single predictor of obesity. Obese individuals ate five grams of dietary fiber less per day than those who were not obese. Individuals who ate 19 or more grams of fiber per day were much less likely to be obese. This fiber can come from vegetables and fruits as well as whole grains. In fact, the most obese subjects in this study ate more fat, less fiber, and fewer complex carbohydrates.

Another fiber-related study, by Harvard Medical School/

Brigham and Women's Hospital, was published in the November 2003 issue of *American Journal of Clinical Nutrition*. It highlights the relationship between choosing whole grains and weight. Data was collected over a twelve-year period from almost seventy-five thousand women aged thirty-eight to sixty-three. The women who ate more whole grains consistently weighed less. Those who consumed the most dietary fiber from whole grains were 49 percent less likely to gain weight than those who ate foods made with refined grains. Weight gain was related to the intake of refined-grain foods, such as white rice and white flour.

The Good Oils: Essential Fatty Acids

Essential fatty acids (EFAs) are oils that are essential to health but cannot be synthesized by the body and so they must come from food. These oils are required to manufacture and repair cell membranes and even to enable the cells to receive nutrition and eliminate toxins. EFAs help to control blood sugar by improving insulin sensitivity, which helps to control weight. Omega-3 EFAs assist in controlling inflammation, which also assists in weight reduction.

The *NBFA* Lifestyle includes plenty of foods rich in essential fatty acids such as flaxseed, flaxseed oil, hempseed, hempseed oil, walnuts, Brazil nuts, sesame seeds, avocados, some dark, leafy green vegetables (kale, spinach, mustard greens, collards), as well as fish oil and fish. Make sure your nuts and seeds are raw since heat and oxygen destroy EFAs.

Add healthy fats to your diet while cutting out bad fats. Flaxseed and hempseed oils are healthy, but never use them for cooking because they can easily oxidize and become toxic. Weight loss is facilitated when you avoid heated oils of all types. However, you can use high-quality extra virgin olive oil, raw coconut oil, or organic ghee with moderate heat.

It's Not Just **What** *You Eat,* *It's* **How** *You Eat*

If you are making the effort to purchase and prepare the best foods, certainly you want to do all you can to gain the greatest possible benefit from them. Here are simple steps you can employ to maximize health, energy, and weight loss.

Overeating is one sure route to self-inflicted misery: lethargy, heaviness, and bloating, not to mention unwanted pounds. The food tastes so good that we eat too much of it. Make it your practice to stop when you have had enough. Much research has concluded that the simplest way to extend your lifespan is by not overeating and even occasionally fasting. The late Dr. Roy Walford, a professor at the UCLA School of Medicine, spent many years researching how to control aging. His studies showed that the one factor that prolongs life is a restricted-calorie diet. Walford was able to double the life span of mice by having them fast two days a week. Not only did these mice live twice as long, but they had significantly less disease.

Once you begin to feed your body nutrient-rich foods, you will need less food (as far as volume is concerned) to be satisfied, since you will be satiated with high-quality, high-fiber foods. Learn to eat what your body needs, rather than what you want. Once unhealthy food addictions are broken, this approach to eating becomes easier.

Overeating is a bad habit that most of us acquire early in life. We eat because it is mealtime, because it tastes good, because we have nothing better to do, because we are depressed, because the social event requires it (or so we think). We eat for so many reasons other than true hunger. Extra food burdens your system. Once you start watching the kinds and amounts of foods you consume, you realize how much unnecessary food is eaten—not only by you, but by nearly everyone in our food-addicted culture. Roe Gallo, in her book *Perfect Body*, writes:

When you feed your body what it needs, your internal fluids stay in balance, your cells are fed, and your body is healthy. Disease, on the other hand, happens when your body is overtaxed, attempting to clean non-nutritious food out of your system. Then your cells starve and eventually die, and so do you. Food that does not directly benefit the body is treated as waste.

Paul Nison, a health writer who healed himself of inflammatory bowel disease, gives this advice in his book *The Raw Life*:

Once you understand that overeating is a bad habit that you must control in order to be in the best of health, you have taken a huge step in the right direction. Anytime you abuse a habit, you form an addiction. Both the habit and the addiction can and must be broken to avoid toxemia. The best way to break a bad habit is with a good habit. Replace the overeating habit with a positive thought and with new healthy habits.

Find hobbies that do not involve eating. Incorporate new activities that cannot be done while you are eating, such as craft projects, home decorating and remodeling, walking, hiking, bicycling, rebounding, or playing a musical instrument. Try to think about something other than food and what you will eat next. Life is more than food and sex, regardless of what the modern media portrays, and the sooner we come to grips with this, the happier and healthier we will be. Remind yourself that if you indulge in the extra food you desire, it will only be in your mouth for seconds or minutes, and afterward you will be sorry. Learn to value your health enough to make these changes.

Nison encourages his readers to avoid overeating by giving the body a break from food for at least twelve to fourteen hours each night. He suggests that we eat only during daylight hours, thus giving our body time to break down all of that food and to rest. One strategy that may help you to stop eating after dinner each evening is to brush and floss your teeth right after the evening meal, while still feeling satisfied. The desire not to repeat this process before bedtime is an encouragement not to eat again. When you go to bed a little on the hungry side, it feels much better than getting into bed full, bloated, and wishing you hadn't overeaten. Your body can then use the sleep time to build and repair, rather than spending the next several hours on the taxing process of digestion.

Another way to avoid overeating is not to skip breakfast. Many people who are trying to lose weight skip breakfast, but it has the opposite effect. Those who don't eat breakfast have an almost five times greater risk of becoming obese. Without having breakfast, you are much more likely to eat more later in the day, whereas breakfast eaters are far less likely to snack. Those who skip breakfast typically eat 40 percent more calories during the day. Moreover, a study cited in the May 2005 issue of *Journal of the American Dietetic Association* reported that eating breakfast seems to "improve cognitive function related to memory, test grades, and school attendance." Kids who eat early in the day are better off in terms of overall nutrition and less likely to be obese. But breakfast is important for all ages, not just children. Studies show that more and more people, especially teenagers, are missing breakfast. People who eat a balanced breakfast weigh less than those who have a sugary one or skip it altogether. If you don't start the day with a nutritious meal, you may refuel midmorning on chocolate, donuts, chips, and other junk foods.

Another approach is to eat several times throughout the day. Eating produces changes in brain chemistry that help to control appetite. Even small changes in the amino acid levels in the blood affect the brain's appetite control center. Snacking is good, but it needs to be with healthy food, not junk food.

Be sure to think positive thoughts and have positive dreams about the healthy person you are becoming. You must envision the healthy, slim person you are becoming and set personal guidelines for yourself (such as deciding you will not eat after the evening meal—unless an out-of-the-ordinary event imposes). These changes won't just happen. You must take control and set these changes in motion.

How to Eat More, but Weigh Less

What would you say if we told you there is a secret that you can employ to enable you to eat more food and still lose weight? Such a strategy does exist. It is not a gimmick, but a method of eating that has scientific support, based on research dating back to the early 1800s. This research was popularized by Dr. William Hay in the 1920s as he discovered that his health improved and his weight dropped substantially within a matter of months simply by eating food in proper combinations that enabled his body to effectively digest. Our ancestors did not combine foods the way that we do. They did not eat hamburgers on buns with French fries or combine grain noodles with cheese, tomatoes, and meat to make lasagna and then top it all off with a peach cobbler dessert. While a variety of foods is desirable, our early ancestors ate their natural foods as they found them, one at a time. If they happened upon a fruit tree, they ate fruit. They did not mix fruit with sugar, oil, and grain to make a pie, nor did they add ice cream to have it à la mode.

Imagine your stomach and the rest of your digestive tract as a test tube, and your food, along with enzymes, as chemicals. Just as wrong combinations in the chemistry lab can result in terrible odors or, even worse, explosions, so it can be in your digestive tract. Wrong combinations in the digestive tract can result in "explosions" such as heartburn, acid reflux, bloating, sharp pains, gas, and constipation, which are the obvious problems, as well as other problems that may go unrecognized. These "hidden" problems stem from undigested food that ferments or putrefies, releasing toxins that poison your entire body. It is a shame to spend money on food but to gain no benefit because you are unable to unlock its nutrients. Poisoning yourself in the process is worse.

Food combining means eating those foods together that require the same chemical environment for their digestion. This approach is dictated by the chemistry of the digestive system, wherein different foods need different enzymes and conditions for their digestion. Very simply, each type of food requires a different combination of digestive juices to be properly digested. Carbohydrates (starches, fruit, and sugar) require a more alkaline environment, while proteins demand a more acidic environment. Whenever you eat foods together that require different environments for digestion, the digestive process is compromised, and the foods may not be properly digested.

Starchy foods, such as grains in any form (bread, pasta, rice, etc.), need an alkaline environment to digest so that the body can break down and use the nutrients they contain. Starches usually are in the stomach for a shorter time than protein. Not only does protein require a longer time in the stomach, it requires a highly acidic environment. In such an acidic environment, the stomach releases pepsin, an enzyme, to digest protein. If you eat both a starch and a protein at the same time, expect problems. As your body pours alkaline components into the digestive system to break down starches and releases acid to digest proteins, the acids and alkalis neutralize each other so that nothing is properly processed. Your valuable digestive enzymes are wasted as more and more are poured into the system to break down this meal of starch along with protein. The body is working so hard that you may feel sluggish. Starches require less time in the stomach before moving on to the intestinal tract, where much of their digestion occurs. When starches enter the stomach with proteins, which require a longer time in the stomach, they get held up. The starch begins to ferment, creating toxins and causing gas, bloating, abdominal discomfort, acid indigestion, poor nutrient absorption, and many other problems. Since most people in our society eat protein along with starch (the meat-and-potatoes diet), no wonder indigestion has become almost normal. (Americans spend more than $2 billion a year on antacids.)

Fruit is another consideration. Fruit inherently contains all of the enzymes necessary for its digestion, so it can and should pass through the system in much less time than either starch or protein. Some fruits, such as melons, are only in the stomach for fifteen to twenty minutes, and others are there slightly longer—but not nearly as long as starch, let alone protein. What happens when you eat a big meal and then have fruit for dessert? Picture the test tube, your stomach, full and mixing in enzymes as it churns the meal. Along comes fruit, which is designed to pass right through, but now it cannot. It is stuck behind the clog in the drainpipe. When fruit is forced to remain in the stomach with a starch, the mixture ferments, creating toxins that spread throughout the body. If the fruit remains in the stomach with a protein meal, digestion is again impaired, and the protein putrefies, similarly resulting in powerful toxins being released into your body. In addition, since you cannot reap the nourishment from most of the food consumed, you are hungry again soon, and your body is crying for nourishment. This causes you to eat more, while toxifying your body—a vicious cycle that is bad for your health and a major obstacle to weight control.

Our digestive systems were not designed to eat what has become our nation's "normal" diet. Many of these foods may still be enjoyed, but learning a new way to eat them will maximize the benefit you receive from them. For example, if you eat three meals a day, have one fruit meal, one starch meal, and one protein meal (not necessarily animal protein). Fruit is a wonderful morning food (as long as you don't have a blood-sugar problem). Since the stomach is empty, fruit can pass right through, and the body can easily absorb and incorporate all of its life-giving vitamins, minerals, trace minerals, and enzymes to make us flourish. Eating fruit in the morning also extends the time the body has to "rest" and eliminate since active digestion is not required. Lunch can be a starch and vegetable meal for which the body readily provides an alkaline environment or a protein and vegetable meal, prompting the system to make an acid environment to allow all of the goodness to be extracted and put to use to replenish and repair cells. You don't feel so sleepy after lunch because the battle within, to digest the meal, does not exist. You feel better because your body is not struggling with an impossible task. You feel energized as your body is able to actually use the nutrients since they have been broken down and can be absorbed. In addition, you are not being poisoned. For dinner, you can eat another meal of starch or protein and vegetables. This makes for optimal digestion, and it is so easy, yet so transforming.

The three guidelines for food combining are as follows:

1. **Eat starches** (such as grains; starchy vegetables such as potatoes, sweet potato, corn, legumes, and beans; pasta; or bread) **with vegetables, but *not* with protein or fruit.**
2. **Eat protein** (such as nuts, seeds, or the small amount of meat or fish you may choose to consume) **with non-starchy vegetables, and *not* with starches.**
3. **Eat fruit alone.** (Acid fruits, such as citrus fruits, apples, mangoes, all berries, cherries, pears, apricots, and peaches may be eaten with raw nuts.)

The recipes in this book, for the most part, adhere to these guidelines. During transition and on special occasions, you won't always live by these guidelines. We realize that there may be times when you are "forced" to eat a poorly combined meal or choose to do so. It may actually prove to be helpful for you to see how it makes you feel. Once you are generally following these rules, you will have more energy (thereby burning more calories), get more nutrients (thereby requiring less food), and will feel better after eating. Many have eliminated their heartburn and acid reflux by following these simple suggestions.

Another reason that our lifestyles have made proper food combining difficult is that we have learned to associate a bloated, full feeling (resulting from a poorly combined meal) with how one is "supposed" to feel after eating. As Marilu Henner suggests in her book *Total Health Makeover*:

> Certain diets purposely miscombine food because they want you to feel somewhat "unresolved." The classic "one bread exchange, one protein exchange, followed by a fruit exchange" approach to dieting was designed to teach people who are used to consuming large amounts of food to eat less by eating smaller portions, yet they'll still feel full. Mixing starch and protein and topping it off with a fruit will definitely make you feel like you've eaten a bigger meal than you have. Ultimately, these diets tend not to work in the long run because your body never gets to experience that really well-digested, cleaned-out feeling that you start to prefer and strive for.

Eat (Chew Well), Drink (Very Little), and Be Merry

An old maxim is that we must remember to chew our food well because there are no teeth in our stomach. In order to maximize health, we must optimize the digestion of all the high-quality foods we consume. Vegetables have a rigid cell wall that must be crushed to unlock life-enhancing nutrients. If this does not occur in your mouth, it will not happen. If it doesn't happen, your cells do not get the nutrition they need, and you feel hungry. Chew your food well—try to see how long you can chew each bite. This lengthens your mealtime and makes the eating process more satisfying. As food is chewed, this crushes the cell walls, releases nutrients, and mixes the food with digestive enzymes that are excreted only in the mouth. Chew your food until it is liquid before you swallow. Unchewed food is usually not digested well and forms toxins. Some people prefer to blenderize or juice their vegetables. This makes even more nutrition available, but the juice must be fresh. Commercial juices are usually pasteurized and too old, have lost too much nutrition, and may contain mold and other toxins.

Another bad habit most people have is drinking too much liquid with their meals. The best way to make the most of the nutrients you consume is not to water down the digestive process. When large amounts of fluid are consumed with a meal, digestive fluids are diluted and are not as effective in breaking down foods. This is one reason that the common practice of indulging in fast food along with a biggie soft drink further inhibits the digestion of a meal that is already a poor food combination. That is not to say that some liquid with a meal is bad. Sipping a glass of organic wine or a similar amount of water is not going to harm, but avoid large amounts.

A good practice is to drink vital, life-giving water between meals rather than with them. Drink a big glass of pure water thirty minutes before your meal; a cup of hot water (coffee temperature) is even better, especially if you do some deep breathing after you drink it. This will actually help to make you less hungry. By incorporating more uncooked food in your meal, you are able to drink less at mealtime. When much of your food is raw vegetables, you do not become as thirsty because they are 70 to 95 percent water. Meals consisting predominantly of cooked food (which has had most of the water cooked out of it) or salty foods create thirst.

What About Water?

A large number of Americans are dehydrated. F. Batmanghelidj wrote an entire manual, *Your Body's Many Cries for Water,* delineating the evidence that many of today's so-called diseases are actually brought on by dehydration. Our bodies are almost 70 percent water by weight. Almost every organ in our body is largely made up of water, and our blood is 83 percent water. Our cells are composed of a nutrient fluid that is mostly water and exist in a saline water environment. In his book, *Water: The Ultimate Cure,* Steve Meyerowitz states that, "If your body's water content drops by as little as 2%, you will feel fatigued. If it drops by 10%, you will experience significant health problems. Losses greater than that can be fatal."

Every ailment from headaches (including migraines), cramps, heartburn, depression, fatigue, constipation, and allergies to fibromyalgia, angina pain, joint pain, hypertension, and autoimmune diseases can be the result of dehydration.

Dehydration is so prevalent that most of us often mistake thirst for hunger. Our bodies are actually thirsty, but we feed them instead, adding unnecessary calories. Having adequate water for our bodies is especially helpful when an individual wants or needs to lose weight. When you feel hungry, try drinking a large glass of water before immediately resorting to food—especially if it is between meals. If you keep yourself well hydrated with fresh pure water, you will eat less, feel fuller, keep your alimentary canal running and, in the long run, lose weight.

Saying that eight, 8-ounce glasses of water per day is the requirement can be misleading. Larger people may require more than that, and smaller individuals may need less. People living in hot, dry climates require more water as well as those who do a lot of physical work. The question of what kind of water to drink will be addressed in chapter 6.

Dedicate Yourself

We have told you up front that this lifestyle requires dedication, but it is worth the effort. Feeling great makes us happy. Eating well makes us look and feel well. We encourage you to begin today to increasingly build your diet around the valuable, nourishing foods we have discussed. Dedicate yourself and your kitchen to health and happiness.

You can still prepare delicious and satisfying meals. The *NBFA* Lifestyle does not require deprivation. The key to keep in mind is to predominantly eat those foods that contain the maximum amount of nutrients for each calorie consumed, which automatically means eating more fresh, unprocessed plant foods (whole fruits, vegetables, legumes, and grains); it is the secret to permanent weight loss and optimal health. There are more and more health restaurants dedicated to serving enticing entrées and desserts that don't contain sugar, white flour, processed oils, dairy, or animal products. You can learn how to do this too. All it takes is determination to change your lifestyle and willingness to learn how.

OTHER PIECES OF THE OVERWEIGHT PUZZLE

5

Y ou are about to be made aware of some common causes of disease and overweight that you probably don't know about. Indeed, if everyone were to pay attention to these causes on a daily basis, most disease would simply disappear. Among the information you'll learn in this chapter:

- How losing weight just to gain it back again damages metabolism and leads to long-term health problems.
- Why deprivation is not the way to be healthy or thin.
- What foods have sodium and how easy it is to get an excess, derailing health and weight loss.
- Which foods are acid forming and which are alkaline, and how this affects your health and weight.

- An imbalance in essential oils is common and keeps you unhealthy and fat.
- The role of hormones for overall health, and how they can inhibit or encourage weight loss.
- Food addictions and allergies are more common than you think, and they can prevent vital health and weight loss.

Diets don't work! They are temporary measures that reap temporary results. . . . Is it fun taking off weight only to put it back on and then repeat the cycle? Do you like measuring portions, counting calories, being deprived, and taking the joy out of the eating experience?

—Harvey Diamond
Fit for Life, Not Fat for Life

After failing with numerous diets and gimmicks, many people give up hope of losing weight. Some end up convincing themselves that their weight is a genetic problem that cannot be solved. "Diets don't work," was the conclusion of Richard, nearly fifty, who was a victim of yo-yo dieting. He began to think his problems were genetic. Although he tried numerous popular diets, including low-calorie starvation diets, low-fat diets, and low-carb diets, he failed to sustain his weight loss. In fact, Richard usually gained back more pounds than he lost. Whenever he started a diet, he often had quick results. His friends would comment, "Wow, you've lost a lot of weight. . . . Bet you feel great!" The problem was that he didn't feel great. He felt worse, and he never understood why.

At six feet and 275 pounds, Richard's obesity was damaging his health, and he felt increasingly fatigued. He ate the typical, nutritionally deficient American diet that fills you with calories and deprives you of essential nutrients. He got little exercise. He was miserable. He suffered one cold after another, severe enough to "knock me out." It was a real labor to climb the stairs to his bedroom, resulting in huffing, puffing, and exhaustion. He looked forward to leaving work and going home to rest. He was prediabetic, suffering from high triglycerides, low levels of "good" HDL cholesterol, high blood pressure, and insulin resistance. He suffered joint pain, muscle cramping, hair loss, skin problems, and short-term memory loss.

Very concerned about his declining health, Richard decided to implement what he had learned to address his mounting health problems—not even thinking about losing weight. Like most people, Richard never thought of his overweight and health problems as having common causes. Richard eagerly adopted the *NBFA* Lifestyle. He cut the toxic Big Four out of his life and added more fresh fruits, vegetables, whole grains, raw nuts, and legumes. Richard worked to lower his toxic load by eating organic foods, eliminating processed foods and artificial sweeteners, and choosing nontoxic personal-care products. He began a program of high-quality nutritional supplements and also purchased a rebounder (mini-trampoline), bouncing on it to improve his lymphatic drainage and detoxification.

Sure enough, it worked. Richard stopped getting colds, his energy soared, his memory improved, his aches and pains gradually went away, and his skin became soft, smooth, and young looking. Life was less a chore and more fun. Richard's mood improved. As his health improved, he started walking to work, and now he even runs up the stairs. He looks much younger. As a happy side effect of his improving health, in the first ten months, he lost fifty-six pounds. Richard surprised himself as well as his friends and coworkers who couldn't believe the miraculous transformation.

Today, Richard's health and weight continue to improve. He feels confident that he has finally discovered a permanent solution to his weight problem, and he wasn't even looking for it. For the first time, he feels great after losing weight. In fact, he felt the health benefits before he noticed the weight loss. Richard has a new lease on life, feeling the best he has ever felt and able to enjoy activities that were formerly impossible for him because of his weight. The *NBFA* Lifestyle will help you, like Richard, to achieve what you may have thought was impossible.

Yo-Yo, Oh No!

Richard had no idea how dangerous yo-yo dieting is. Rapid weight loss, undertaken without considering overall health, interferes with natural weight control mechanisms, leading to unnatural and even dangerous eating patterns that ultimately fail. Richard achieved speedy reductions in weight by drastically reducing calories or cutting out an entire category of nutrients, such as fat, carbohydrates, or protein. Meanwhile, he continued to eat fake processed foods loaded with toxic additives, sugar, and artificial sweeteners. This is not a recipe for long-term health. Rather than cutting out a class of nutrients or a radical change in caloric intake, what is required is eating more nutrient- and fiber-rich whole foods that are filling and satisfying and automatically lower in calories, along with an increase in physical activity. Eating fewer calories than those required to maintain normal weight causes your body to dehydrate, losing water and leading to rapid weight loss. You may think you want this, but you don't. Eating too few calories sets off biological alarm bells. The body thinks it is starving and tells you to eat more. After the dehydration phase, you start to lose muscle mass. About half of the weight loss is muscle, but when weight is regained almost all of it is fat. Since muscles burn fat, about seventy times as much as fat cells, having less muscle tissue decreases fat burning, preserves fat, and makes it easier to gain fat later on. *This is how dieting makes you fat.* This vicious cycle happens to a lot of yo-yo dieters, as it did to Richard.

Yo-yo dieting is detrimental to health and makes you gain weight because you keep losing fat-burning muscle and gaining back more fat. People on such diets actually make themselves fatter and sicker. It is also psychologically discouraging to keep losing the same weight over and over again, while gaining back even more. A 2004 study reported in the *Journal of the American Dietetic Association* found that the more times you lose and regain weight by dieting, the more long-term damage is done to your immune system. Natural killer cell (a special type of immune cell that targets tumors and protects against a wide variety of infectious microbes) activity becomes depressed, making you more susceptible to cancer and infections. Yo-yo dieters are also at higher risk for heart disease. A 2000 study reported in the *Journal of the American College of Cardiology* found that dieters who habitually lose and regain weight have lower levels of the healthy HDL cholesterol.

Statistics show that most people who go on popular low-calorie diet plans regain their lost pounds within one year, and only a tiny percentage do not regain the unwanted pounds within five years. At any one time, about one out of three Americans is on a diet, but only one out of five stays on that diet for more than a month. Amazingly, one out of three dieters actually gains weight while they are trying to lose it. This fact alone reveals that diets are ineffective.

Don't Deprive Yourself

Your body's innate intelligence tries to protect you from starvation and harm. When you take in less than the necessary building blocks to maintain the physical body, the body interprets this situation as starvation and begins to consume its own tissue to stay alive. In alarm, your body believes it is starving and intensifies food cravings and food-seeking behavior. If the body fails to get you to eat more, metabolism slows in order to reduce the number of calories burned and conserve energy, thus burning less fat. So the fat stays right where it is, and, in fact, fat storage is increased. *When you go off the low-calorie diet, although you begin taking in more calories, you will still be burning fewer calories, because the body does not quickly reset its metabolic rate.* You are worse off than you were in the first place. You gain the lost weight back—often gaining more than you lost.

Opinions differ about how many calories are needed for normal weight and functioning. On average, you need fifteen calories for every pound of your ideal body weight; however, that amount differs widely from person to person depending on genes, weight, age, sex, metabolic rate, and physical activity. For example, some athletes consume four thousand calories per day. A physically active teenage male might need thirty-five hundred calories, while a small, inactive older woman might do well at sixteen hundred. Particularly when consuming fewer calories, it becomes especially important that every calorie be nutrient-rich.

Although men lose weight faster than women, and larger people faster than smaller, as a rule of thumb, if you are losing more than two pounds per week, you are going too fast. *Two pounds per week or even less is plenty.* Remember that the excess weight was not added in a matter of days or weeks, and you should not expect to lose it that way either. Findings in medical literature indicate that rapid weight loss is much harder to sustain.

Calorie-restrictive diets have been found to have other serious health consequences, including increased risk of diabetes, gallstones, stroke, cognitive impairment, and premature death. The best way to handle this problem is to never starve yourself of essential nutrients. Eat plenty of real food—fresh fruits, vegetables, whole grains, raw nuts, and legumes. Real food supplies adequate calories and lots of nutrients and fiber to make you feel full, eliminating the desire for excess calories.

Portions Out of Control

Limiting ourselves to eating only what we need is still a challenge. Part of Richard's problem was societal. He got caught up in a society where instant gratification, driven by advertising and consumerism, has elevated excess to a cultural art form—the "Super-Size Me" era. As the nutrients per calorie in most modern food are decreasing, the portion size has been steadily increasing. Increasing portion size is one of the factors responsible for the epidemic of overweight disease. From 1971 to 1998, the average soft-drink increased from thirteen ounces with 144 calories to twenty ounces with 193 calories. Salty snacks grew from 1-ounce bags to 1.6-ounce bags and from 132 to 225 calories. In the winter of 2004–2005, Starbucks started offering a new hot chocolate drink called the Chantico—it has 390 calories. Hardee's Monster Thickburger has 1,420 calories! That's a lot of calories. Not surprisingly, from 1985 to 2000, daily calorie consumption in the United States increased by 300 calories per day, while physical activity decreased.

Another unfortunate trend, nutrient-poor foods comprise an ever-greater proportion of the American diet. A June 2004 study reported in the *Journal of Food Chemistry and Analysis* concluded that sweets, soft drinks, and alcohol make up one-quarter of all the calories consumed by Americans—all empty calories devoid of nutrition. Salty snacks and fruit-flavored drinks make up another 5 percent, bringing the calories from nutrient-poor junk foods to at least 30 percent of total calorie intake. To supply cells with all that they need to be healthy, every calorie needs to be filled with nutrients—eating worthless junk is not an option.

Sugar, the wrong fats, and nutrient deficiency have all been shown to artificially stimulate the appetite. Put them together as junk foods, and it is no wonder that we have become a nation of fatties craving larger and larger portions. The

challenge is to remove junk foods and other sugary, fatty, and
nutrient-deficient foods from your life and replace them with
nutrient-rich whole foods.

Common Causes of
Cellular Malfunction, Disease, and Weight Gain

The reasons you gain weight and have trouble losing weight
are varied, but four play a key role. They are fundamental to
maintaining your cellular health and avoiding disease, including overweight. Take control of these, and you will succeed.
Ignore them at your peril. These health-building keys are:

- the ratio between sodium and potassium in your cells
- the balance in your body between acid and alkaline
  environments
- adequate intake of essential fatty acids
- the amount of inflammation you create in your system

Other factors—including hormones, food addictions, and
allergies—play important roles in weight control. However, the
sodium/potassium ratio, acid-alkaline balance, essential fatty
acids, and inflammation are so fundamental to healthy cell
function that we have helped numerous clients to lose weight,
and to reduce and even reverse heart disease, cancer, diabetes,
arthritis, osteoporosis, Alzheimer's disease, and other chronic
diseases, by teaching them how to control these factors. This
could not be more simple or more powerful. If you do things
right in each of these areas—*and you can*—you will go a long
way toward preventing or reversing almost any disease.

Too Much Sodium

Common table salt (sodium chloride) is a leading cause of
disease because excess sodium causes cells to malfunction.
Sodium and potassium are minerals that are critical to cell

function, but they must be properly balanced. Modern dietary practices create serious imbalances. Our ancestors consumed low-sodium, high-potassium diets. Their sodium/potassium ratio was a healthy 1 to 4, the result of eating plenty of potassium-rich fresh fruits and vegetables. Our current ratio is reversed to an unhealthy 4 to 1, because we are eating sodium-rich processed foods and insufficient fruits and vegetables.

Cells function like little batteries. Cells have an electrical charge created by the difference in the amount of potassium inside the cell and the amount of sodium outside. Your cell batteries supply the electricity that causes your heart to beat and your brain to function. By consuming excess dietary sodium we change the sodium/potassium ratio in our cells, which damages the "battery of life" and interferes seriously with the body's self-regulation and repair functions, sapping your energy and making you feel run down and tired.

On average, the human body requires only about 220 milligrams (mg) of sodium per day. A teaspoon of regular refined salt contains about 2,300 mg of sodium. *We recommend no more than 1,000 mg of sodium per day, or a little less than a half teaspoon.* (In special circumstances, such as excessive sweating or diarrhea, higher levels may be necessary.)

Achieving a goal of 1,000 mg per day is not that difficult. Just cut out processed foods, and be careful where you eat and what you order when you eat out. About 10 percent of the sodium in the American diet is found naturally in food; about 10 to 15 percent is added as table salt, and the remaining 75 to 80 percent comes from processed, packaged foods. The refined salt in commercially processed foods causes most of our sodium/potassium imbalance. Due to our consumption of processed foods, most Americans ingest 4,000 to 7,000 mg of sodium per day, and many are exposed to as much as 10,000 to 20,000 mg per day. Processors add salt to enhance flavor, mask bad flavors, preserve color, and modify the texture of a food. The more highly processed a food is, the more likely it is to have a high sodium content.

Here's an example of how easy it is to get too much sodium. The following nutritional information was obtained from a popular soup-and-salad restaurant chain. If you have a bowl of their split-pea soup, you will consume 1,430 mg of sodium. Choosing a couple of the salad offerings adds another 400 mg. A serving of their "healthy" nonfat Italian salad dressing adds another 1,350 mg. Two "healthy" low-fat muffins add another 1,400 mg. This "healthy" lunch of soup, salad, and low-fat muffins adds up to a whopping 4,580 mg of sodium. This is more sodium than you should have in almost five days—at just one meal! To balance your cell chemistry with potassium from just this one meal, you would need to eat sixteen bananas. Overdosing on sodium is surprisingly easy.

When your sodium intake is too high, your bones can weaken. For every 2,000 mg of salt you eat, you will lose about 23 mg of calcium in your urine. Unless you replace these calcium losses, and most people don't eat enough bioavailable calcium to fully replace them all, then eating an average of 5,000 mg of sodium per day could result in losses as high as 2.5 percent of your skeleton annually for a total of 25 percent in only ten years—one reason that so many older people have weak bones and suffer from osteoporosis. Also, because sodium helps to regulate the amount of water both inside and outside of cells, an excess causes water retention, which increases weight.

In June 2006, the American Medical Association (AMA) voted to petition the government to require high-salt foods to be labeled. The AMA said there is overwhelming evidence that excessive salt is a risk factor for disease. It urged the food and restaurant industries to drastically cut the amount of salt in processed and restaurant food by 50 percent within a decade. It also called for the Food and Drug Administration to remove salt from the list of foods "generally recognized as safe." The AMA should have done this decades ago, but better late than never. However, don't wait for the government to take action, which may be long in coming. Protect yourself and your family—now.

Cellular pH: Acidity Interferes with Fat Burning

The degree of acidity or alkalinity is expressed as "pH." Abnormal cellular pH is another common denominator of cellular malfunction, disease, and overweight. Cells malfunction when their pH is wrong because critical chemical reactions in the body are dependent upon chemicals called enzymes. However, enzymes function in a narrow pH range. If your cells change their pH for any reason, enzymes are disabled and many critical chemical reactions will not take place. Most Americans are too acidic, and too much acidity inhibits fat-burning enzymes, contributing to overweight.

The pH scale runs from 0 to 14, with 7.0 being neutral, 0 the most acidic, and 14 the most alkaline. Normal cellular pH is slightly alkaline at about 7.42. When cellular pH becomes too acidic, cells malfunction and bodily systems are weakened, creating an environment in which disease becomes inevitable. Healthy bodies are equipped with alkaline reserves that can be utilized to neutralize excess acids. When our diet regularly consists of acid-forming foods (which the Standard American Diet does), our reserves are depleted and we become vulnerable not only to weight gain, premature aging, and low energy, but also to cancer, cardiovascular damage, diabetes, osteoporosis, immune deficiency, and organ malfunction of every kind. Even a small degree of acidity can lead to fatigue and feeling generally subpar. Acidic cells lower your metabolic rate, preventing fat from being burned. In his book *The pH Miracle,* author Robert Young had this to say:

Food & Chemical Effects on Acid

Most Akaline	More Alkaline	Low Alkaline	Lowest Alkaline
Baking Soda	Spices/Cinnamon	Herbs (most); Arnica	White Willow Bark
	Valerian	Bergamot, Echinacea	Slippery Elm
	Licorice	Chrysanthemum,	Artemesia Annua
	Black Cohosh	Epedra, Feverfew,	
	Agave	Goldenseal, Lemongrass	
		Aloe Vera	
		Nettle	
		Angelica	
Sea Salt			*Sulfite*
Mineral Water	Kambucha	Green or Mu Tea	Ginger Tea
	Molasses	Rice Syrup	Sucanat
	Soy Sauce	Apple Cider Vinegar	Umeboshi Vinegar
Umeboshi Plum		Sake	Algae, Blue Green
			Ghee (Clarified Butter)
			Human Breast Milk
		Quail Egg	Duck Egg
			Oat
			Grain Coffee
			Quinoa
			Wild rice
			Japonica Rice
	Poppy Seed	Primrose Oil	Avocado Oil
Pumpkin Seed	Cashew	Sesame Seed	Seeds (most)
	Chestnut	Cod Liver Oil	Coconut Oil
	Pepper	Almond	Olive/Macadamia Oil
Hydrogenated Oil		Sprout	Linseed/Flax Oil
Lentil	Kohlrabi	Potato/Bell Pepper	Brussels Sprout
Brocoflower	Parsnip/Taro	Mushroom/Fungi	Beet
Seaweed	Garlic	Cauliflower	Chive/Cilantro
Noril/Kombu/Wakame/Hijiki	Asparagus	Cabbage	Celery/Scallion
Onion/Miso	Kale/Parsley	Rutabaga	Okra/Cucumber
Daikon/Taro Root	Endive/Arugula	Salsify/Ginseng	Turnip Greens
Sea Vegetables (other)	Mustard Greens	Eggplant	Squash
Dandelion Green	Jerusalem Artichoke	Pumpkin	Artichoke
Burdock/Lotus Root	Ginger Root	Collard Greens	Lettuce
Sweet Potato/Yam	Broccoli		Jicama
Lime	Grapefruit	Lemon	Orange
Nectarine	Canteloupe	Pear	Apricot
Persimmon	Honeydew	Avocado	Banana
Raspberry	Citrus	Apple	Blueberry
Watermelon	Olive	Blackberry	Pineapple Juice
Tangerine	Dewberry	Cherry	Raisin, Currant
Pineapple	Loganberry	Peach	Grape
	Mango	Papaya	Strawberry

Italicized items are NOT recommended

kaline Body Chemical Balance

Food Category	Lowest Acid	Low Acid	More Acid	Most Acid
Spice/Herb	Curry	Vanilla Stevia	*Nutmeg*	Pudding/Jam/Jelly
Preservative	*MSG*	*Benzoate*	*Aspartame*	*Table Salt (NaCL)*
Beverage	*Kona Cofee*	*Alcohol* Black Tea	*Coffee*	Beer, *Soda* Yeast/Hops/Malt
Sweetner	Honey/Maple Syrup		*Saccharin*	Sugar/Cocoa
Vinegar	Rice Vinegar	Balsamic Vinegar	Red Wine Vinegar	White/Acetic Vinegar
Therapeutic		*Antihistamines*	*Psychotropics*	*Antibiotics*
Processed dairy	Cream/Butter	Cow Milk	Casein, Milk Protein, Cottage Cheese	*Processed Cheese*
Cow/Human	Yogurt	Aged Cheese	New Cheese	Ice Cream
Soy		Soy Cheese	Soy Milk	
Goat/Sheep	Goat/sheep Cheese	Goat Milk		
Egg	Chicken Egg			
Meat	Gelatin/Organs	Lamb/Mutton	Pork/Veal	Beef
Game	Venison	Boar/Elk/Game Meat	Bear	
Fish/Shell Fish	Fish	Shell Fish/Mollusks	Mussel/Squid	Lobster
Fowl	Wild Duck	Goose/Turkey	Chicken	Pheasant
Grain Cereal Grass	Triticale Millet Kasha Amaranth Brown Rice	Buckwheat Wheat Spelt/Teff/Kamut Farina/Semolina White Rice	Maize Barley Groat Corn Rye Oat Bran	Barley *Processed Flour*
Nut Seed/Sprout Oil	Pumpkin Seed Oil Grape Seed Oil Sunflower Oil Pine Nut Canola Oil	Almond Oil Sesame Oil Safflower Oil Tapioca Seitan or Tofu	Pistachio Seed Chestnut Oil *Lard* Pecan Palm kernel Oil	*Cottonseed Oil/Meal* Hazelnut Walnut Brazil Nut *Fried Food*
Bean Vegetable Legume Pulse Root	Spinach Fava Bean Kidney Bean Black-eyed Pea String/Wax Bean Zucchini Chutney Rhubarb	Split Pea Pinto Bean Whilte Bean Navy/Red Bean Aduki Bean Lima or Mung Bean Chard	Green Pea Peanut Snow Pea Legumes (other) Carrot Chick Pea/Garbanzo	Soybean Carob
Citrus Fruit Fruit	Coconut Guava Pickled Fruit Dry Fruit Fig Persimmon Juice Cherimoya Date	Plum Prune Tomato	Cranberry Pomegranate	

You can thank an overly acid internal environment for the excess pounds you are carrying around. In a defensive maneuver, the body creates fat cells to carry acids away from your vital organs to try to protect them. In one sense, your fat is saving your life! But that's why your body doesn't want to let it go. When you eat to make your body more basic [alkaline], your body won't need to keep the fat anymore.

Where is all this excess acidity coming from? Primarily from a diet high in acid-forming foods such as meat, eggs, dairy, white flour, sugar, coffee, chemical sweeteners, fruit drinks, and soft drinks (notice that these are all foods excluded from the *NBFA* Lifestyle). Colas combine sugar with phosphoric acid, producing a powerful acidic effect. Acidity also comes from stress. Any kind of stress, physical or emotional, tends to acidify your body, including the biochemical stress created by illness and allergic reactions. Stress combined with acid foods compounds the problem. Fresh fruits and vegetables generally make your pH more alkaline, as do sleep, meditation, and other forms of relaxation, and an adequate intake of minerals. The table on pages 122 and 123 shows the acidity/alkalinity of different foods.

You can measure your own pH at home by testing your first morning urine after at least six hours of bed rest. (See Appendix D for pH testing paper.) To do the test, tear off about an inch and a half of paper from the roll and pass it through your urine stream. The yellow pH paper will change color. A chart that comes with the pH paper matches colors with numbers. Your urine pH reading should be between 6.5 and 7.5; an ideal range would be 6.8 to 7.4. (Although testing throughout the day is interesting—you can see immediate reactions to various foods and activities—first morning pH most closely approximates what is happening inside your cells.)

If you are eating an alkalinizing diet and your pH is still too acidic, work to identify and eliminate any allergies (an allergic reaction can cause acidity for several days), reduce stress, and see Appendix D for a protocol for using supplemental magnesium to balance pH.

The Right Fats Are Essential

We discussed earlier that each cell has a wall called the cell membrane that is largely composed of fats. To prevent and reverse disease, the billions of new cells we create every day must be constructed with the right fats, in the correct proportions.

Unfortunately for us, the processed vegetable and hydrogenated oils that predominate our diet are the wrong building materials and create faulty cell membranes. Most of the oils consumed today are toxic. Almost every oil and every oil-containing product (which is almost all packaged foods) you purchase in a supermarket is toxic. These processed oils are deficient in omega-3 fats and contain trans fats, oxidized fats, and excessive omega-6s. An estimated 95 percent of Americans are deficient in omega-3 fats. This deficiency has led to an epidemic of suboptimal and deteriorating health, including diseases such as cardiovascular disease, cancer, multiple sclerosis, and diabetes.

The major reason for this deficiency of omega-3s is the massive switch during the twentieth century from traditional fats and oils to hydrogenated and processed vegetable oils. Another reason is changes in livestock feeding. Traditionally fed only on grass, livestock on commercial farms today are fed grain in order to increase their fat and weight. Cattle fed on grass will have an omega-6 to omega-3 ratio of approximately 3 to 1, whereas today's grain-fed beef has ratios of 20 to 1 and higher. (Also, grass-fed beef has far less total body fat and far less saturated fat. About 10 percent of their fat will be saturated compared with up to 50 percent for the grain-fed.)

If you purchase beef, and we recommend very little of that, you should ensure that the "grass-fed" beef you are buying is also "grass-finished." All cows eat grass in the early part of their lives. The grain feeding occurs in feedlots where cows are fattened up prior to slaughter. As consumer demand for grass-fed beef has grown, some unscrupulous beef suppliers are claiming their beef is "grass fed" even though it has been grain finished.

Chickens once dined on insects, earthworms, and weeds, and their eggs were excellent sources of omega-3s. But now it is the rare chicken that gets to eat its preferred food, and commercially produced eggs are poor sources of omega-3s. Try to find farmers in your area who allow their chickens to feed freely on what nature provides. The yolks of these eggs will be orange-yellow, the darker orange the better. In addition to doing your part to support the humane treatment of chickens (most commercial chicken farms are anything but humane, and chickens are apt to be sickly as well as low on omega-3s), you will be consuming eggs from healthy poultry, which is absolutely healthier for you. "Free range" is not enough. This is merely a guarantee that the chickens have some room to move around in their pens. Also "organic" is not enough. Organic means only that chickens are being fed organic grain. However, organic is often the best choice available, depending on where you live.

Although fish have been prized as a remaining source of omega-3s, more and more fish are now being raised on farms where they are being fed grain. This unnatural food source produces fish with fewer omega-3s and a less favorable balance of fats.

Whenever possible, buy wild-caught fish. Farmed fish also contains more toxins and should be avoided for that reason alone.

Our cell walls need a minimum of about 3 grams of omega-3 fats a day. You can get 3 grams from half a tablespoon of flax oil or one tablespoon of cod-liver oil. However, unless you have been going out of your way to obtain omega-3s from fish or flax, you are probably deficient and should take at least twice this amount in order to replenish your body's stores. The most recent evidence suggests that once the body's omega-6 to omega-3 ratio becomes imbalanced with too much omega-6, it can take years to restore a more appropriate balance.

Take a tablespoon each of cod-liver and flax oil daily, which together supply 7.5 grams of omega-3 fats. Each oil provides unique health benefits in addition to supplying omega-3 fats. Handle these oils with care. Omega-3s are very perishable. Make sure your oils are as fresh as possible, and keep the bottles refrigerated—frozen when you are not using them.

In addition to the task of building healthy cell membranes, the ratio of omega-6 to omega-3 oils in your diet is significant in other ways as well. Omega-6 oils are inflammatory, and omega-3 oils have the opposite, anti-inflammatory effect, which plays an important role in chronic inflammatory diseases and overweight.

Inflammation Wreaks Havoc

Inflammation is a common factor in all chronic disease, including overweight. A major reason we have so much disease in our society is that we have so much inflammation. A major reason for this inflammation is our inflammatory diet. Controlled inflammation is both natural and healing. For example, if you cut your finger, the body immediately begins an inflammatory process. This process neutralizes harmful microorganisms, helps to repair the wound, and cleans up the debris resulting from the injury. Inflammation is beneficial when needed, but it is disastrous when chronic.

What causes chronic inflammation? The Standard American Diet. We suffer from chronic inflammation and disease because the American diet is pro-inflammatory: rich in pro-inflammatory chemicals, while lacking in nutrients that help to prevent and control inflammation. To help reverse this, get the Big Four and all processed foods out of your life.

More than three out of four Americans suffer from diseases of chronic inflammation. Like a fire out of control, chronic inflammation generates a constant supply of free radicals. These overwhelm our antioxidant defenses, destroy healthy cells and tissues, damage DNA, age us, and cause disease of every description, including heart disease, cancer, diabetes, osteoporosis, arthritis, allergies, Alzheimer's disease, autoimmune disease, infections, and overweight.

The inflammatory process can be self-sustaining unless you shut it off with antioxidants. A free radical is a molecule with an unpaired electron. Because electrons like to travel in pairs, a free radical is always looking to steal an electron away from another molecule. After it steals an electron, the original free radical is neutralized. But by depriving a second molecule of its electron partner, it has created a new, highly reactive free radical, which is now frantically seeking to steal an electron from yet another molecule. In this way, a free radical can initiate a damaging chain reaction that keeps the inflammatory process going. In a healthy body, antioxidant reserves keep inflammation in check. Antioxidants are molecules that can comfortably donate an extra electron, and they can nip in the bud a potentially disruptive cascade of free-radical chemical reactions. However, in a condition of chronic inflammation, antioxidant reserves are exhausted, and free radical damage wreaks havoc, destroying and aging body tissues.

Chronic inflammation increases insulin resistance, which leads to higher insulin levels; higher insulin leads to more free radicals, while signaling cells to accumulate fat. With our cells being instructed to store fat, it is easy to gain it and difficult to lose it, unless the underlying chronic inflammation is addressed by reducing the intake of inflammatory foods and increasing the intake of antioxidants. Chronic inflammation also contributes to overweight by causing leptin resistance. Leptin is a hormone that regulates appetite. Leptin helps you feel full, prevents carbohydrate cravings, and tells the body whether to store or release fat. When the body has had enough to eat, leptin suppresses the appetite and stimulates fat burning. When inflammation causes leptin resistance, this reduces leptin's ability to deliver proper appetite and weight-control signals, and the result is fat storage rather than burning. Since fat cells produce inflammatory chemicals, as you gain weight, there is more inflammation, which causes more leptin resistance. More leptin resistance leads to adding more fat, more inflammation, and then more leptin resistance in a vicious cycle. Yet another mechanism by which inflammation can cause weight gain is that inflammatory mediators, such as histamine, can increase capillary permeability, thus causing leakage of water into tissues.

Given the above, to improve health and reduce weight, an anti-inflammatory diet and anti-inflammatory supplements are essential. Here are some things you need to do:

- Eat lots of fresh fruits and vegetables, especially the colorful ones, which have many anti-inflammatory vitamins, minerals, and phytonutrients.
- Get off the Big Four—they are all inflammatory.
- Eliminate dairy products, drastically reduce animal protein, and consume fewer processed grains.
- Get toxins out of your life as much as you can (see chapter 6).
- Favor anti-inflammatory or neutral fats (such as the omega-3s, raw nuts and seeds, and raw coconut and extra virgin olive oil) over the inflammatory fats.
- Avoid rapid elevations of blood sugar from eating refined carbohydrates.
- Avoid highly refined foods of any type because they strain the body as nutrients are robbed from other sources to process them.
- Reduce and/or learn to manage stress. Stress is inflammatory.

- Eliminate chronic infections.
- Get enough sleep. (Sleep deprivation can increase inflammatory markers 40 to 60 percent.)
- Get regular exposure to moderate sunlight.
- Lose weight by adopting the *NBFA* Lifestyle. Fat cells are pro-inflammatory, especially those that accumulate in the abdominal area.
- Take anti-inflammatory supplements such as vitamins A, C, and E as well as other antioxidants including coenzyme Q_{10}, N-acetylcysteine, alpha-lipoic acid, beta carotene, curcumin, quercitin, and selenium. You will learn more about supplements in chapter 11.

Hormones, Allergies, and Addictions Take a Toll

Malnutrition and excess calories are at the heart of overweight disease, but a number of complex factors can play a role. Some individuals have never had success on any diet, which may be because of other factors, such as hormones, addictions, and allergies that can hinder weight loss.

Hormones

If your metabolism slows down while caloric intake remains the same, you will gain weight. The thyroid gland regulates your metabolic speed. If thyroid hormone levels drop and you become hypothyroid, cells throughout the body slow their activity. Hence, people with low thyroid levels often gain weight because they are burning fewer calories.

According to Richard Shames and Karilee Shames, authors of *Thyroid Power: Ten Steps to Total Health,* there is a "runaway epidemic" of hypothyroidism in this country, often undiagnosed because thyroid testing is inadequate, with mild thyroid failure showing up in about 10 percent of the general population and in up to 20 percent of older women, especially postmenopausal women.

We can think of several reasons for this epidemic. One is widespread malnutrition. Numerous nutrients are required to support healthy thyroid function, and function is impaired without them. In addition, the thyroid withdraws thyroid hormone from circulation if it perceives starvation. It does this in order to preserve precious resources. The starvation message can come from a calorie-laden but nutritionally deficient processed-food diet or from low-calorie weight-loss diets, which is one reason that people on low-calorie diets can gain weight.

Another widespread cause is environmental toxicity. Toxic exposure to fluoride (in water, food, and toothpaste) is a major problem that impairs thyroid function. Xenoestrogens (chemicals that have an estrogen-like effect on the body) from fertilizers, pesticides, and plastics are throwing our hormone systems out of balance.

Estrogen excess impedes thyroid function. Since fat cells produce excess estrogen, being overweight can lead to gaining even more weight due to thyroid hormone suppression—a vicious cycle. Estrogen dominance is a hormone issue for many women and even men: having too much estrogen relative to the hormone progesterone in women or testosterone in men. Sometimes, to break this cycle, it may be advisable to use progesterone cream. This should be done under the supervision of a knowledgeable health practitioner. We recommend the conservative approach of trying a good diet and avoiding toxins first—certainly avoiding the toxic hormones found in commercially bred animal proteins and the xenoestrogens from the pesticides in nonorganic produce.

Physicians usually prescribe thyroid hormone supplementation. In some cases this may be unavoidable, but the true solution is to get well by eating a good diet and avoiding dangerous toxins like fluoride (we tell you how to avoid fluoride in chapter 6).

Insight into the role hormones play in the epidemic of overweight children was reported in the June 2005 issue of *Cell Metabolism*. Overweight people have higher levels of the fat-regulating hormone leptin due to leptin resistance, just as diabetics have higher levels of insulin due to insulin resistance. Remember that leptin controls how fat is burned and causes us to feel full. The fetus of an overweight mother is exposed to higher leptin levels, and this exposure early in life appears to change the circuitry in the brain. The brain becomes less sensitive to signals from leptin (leptin resistance), so you don't feel full as readily and fat is not burned as it ought to be. Offspring of malnourished mothers also have problems with leptin. In one study, they stored 50 percent more fat on a high-fat diet compared to those with well-nourished mothers. Individuals born to mothers who were both overweight and malnourished have to be extra careful to adhere to the *NBFA* Lifestyle in order to stay slim.

Addiction and Food Allergies

Most overweight people are addicted to food, and one reason weight-loss diets don't work is that they fail to address addictions. Addictions make it much easier to gain weight and substantially more difficult to lose it. Popular diet plans include allergens, and none exclude all three of the most common allergens: gluten, dairy, and sugar. *When excess calories are the problem, addictions and allergies help supply those calories.*

Simple carbohydrates such as sugar and white flour are known to increase blood insulin, but they do a lot of other things as well, such as increase serotonin (a natural mood upper) and endorphins (nature's natural painkillers). Endorphins result in the sense of euphoria called "runner's high" after prolonged exercise. Serotonin makes you feel good, and lack of it causes depression, sleep problems, aggressiveness, and even violence and suicides.

Life is full of little pains and aggravations, and sugar and other simple carbohydrates can provide a quick fix of pleasure-enhancing serotonin and painkilling endorphins, but the fix is only temporary. Maintaining high levels of these feel-good chemicals requires constant consumption of sugar and white flour. When serotonin is constantly high, the body tries to regulate it by reducing serotonin production. Reduced serotonin production causes depression, so you have to eat more sugar and white flour to get more serotonin in order to maintain normal mood levels. With time, as occurs with street drugs, higher and higher amounts of carbs are needed to get the same effect. More carbs means more calories, and more calories mean more pounds.

Another addiction is dependence on an outside source of glucose. Glucose is used as a fuel to create energy in our cells. This molecule is so important that the body makes its own. However, when we eat a high-carb diet, we strip the body of essential minerals required by the enzymes that manufacture the glucose, and the cells that are used to make the glucose suffer from disuse, creating a situation where we become physically dependent on an outside source.

Allergic reactions to foods are far more common than most people believe, and they can cause cravings and addictions. The term "addictive food allergy" has been suggested to describe the relationship between compulsive eating and allergy. Distress to body tissues caused by allergic reactions promotes the release of powerful painkillers and soothing chemicals to ease the pain and discomfort. Opiumlike chemicals called opioid peptides are released, and these feel-good chemicals are addictive. Any amount of allergens in the diet can trigger such a reaction, which is why it is so important to avoid them completely.

Unconsciously your body craves the allergic foods to provide it with more of the opium-like chemicals, resulting in excessive eating. Instead of making you feel bad, the allergic reaction makes you feel better. As you continue to eat these reactive foods, the stress to the body can actually give you the illusion of increased energy. It's ironic that the foods you long for most are usually the ones to which you are, unbeknownst to you, allergic and addicted. Ultimately, such reactions sap your energy by depleting you of essential nutrients and putting a burden on the body to clean up all the debris from the damage. Low energy is often a symptom of gluten intolerance, and people often turn to caffeine and other stimulants to get through the day.

As if getting too many calories is not bad enough, allergic reactions often result in water retention, which contributes to weight gain. Allergic reactions also lead to an abnormally acidic pH. Overall, this "feel-good" state comes at a very high price—accelerated aging, more disease, overweight, and early death.

The Whole Picture

To get well and stay well, which includes achieving and maintaining your ideal weight, you cannot focus on only one or a few pieces of the puzzle. All the pieces must come together to create the whole picture—your own unique picture of natural health and beauty! It may take more initial effort to understand and master each of the factors involved, but isn't this a better use of your time and effort than going on a series of incomplete, unhealthy diets that ultimately fail? How much better to have a reliable foundation in place through an understanding of what is necessary to accomplish your goal.

PART III

Other Important Weapons for the *NBFA* Lifestyle

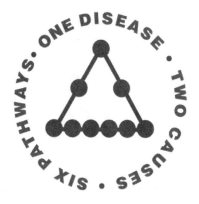

M any diet books tell you what to eat and which foods to avoid and stop there. But nutrition represents just one weapon in your armory, and you cannot win the battle against fat with just one weapon. That is why the section you are about to read sets this book apart from "diet books."

Consider the other weapons—the five additional pathways to health and weight loss: How often have you been shown how toxins in your food, home, and environment can make you fat? You are about to learn how this happens. Did you know that your mind is one of the most powerful weapons in the arsenal for battling extra pounds? It may be the most critical tactic of all, and we show practical ways to employ it for weight loss. The fact that exercise is essential to a healthy, slim lifestyle is not really a surprise, but you may be unaware that there are other practices in the physical realm that can be instrumental for maximizing cellular health and maintaining normal weight. Much is said about the genetic tendency to overweight, but in this part of the book, you learn that you can control the expression of fat genes. You also gain the tools needed to wisely choose or refuse medical interventions along with helpful information about natural supplementation and how to find supplements that truly nourish cells and stimulate weight loss.

THE TOXIN PATHWAY

A critical key to a healthier lifestyle is avoiding toxins, one of the two causes of all disease. In this chapter, you will learn the sources of your toxic exposures, internal and external, and how to avoid or at least minimize most of them. In this chapter, we will discuss:

- What toxins have to do with weight.
- Which chemical food additives are most toxic and why.
- Which foods put you at the highest risk.
- How packaging and preparing foods can make them toxic.
- What genetically modified foods are and why they are dangerous.
- What the hazards in drinking water are and how to avoid them.
- How breathing can make you unhealthy and fat.

- What kinds of toxins are in personal-care and household products.
- The secret tool for releasing toxins while burning fat and calories.

Weight gain is not just down to weak willpower, greed and laziness. Much of it is due to your body's inability to deal with toxins in your food and environment.

—Pamela Baillie-Hamilton
Toxic Overload

One of the critical factors that people trying to lose weight most often miss is how common environmental toxins—from chemicals in food, toiletries, and even in their homes—stand in the way of weight-loss success. Toxins interfere with your appetite-control and fat-management functions. They can keep your appetite turned on while instructing your cells to store fat. Simply put—*environmental toxins may be helping you to pack on the pounds!* If these chemicals are jamming your fat-control system, losing weight will be difficult until you lose the chemicals.

Most of the man-made chemicals to which you are exposed are capable of affecting your weight, at least to some degree, even at extremely low concentrations. Failure to address the role of toxicity is an important reason that weight-loss programs usually fail to deliver lasting success. Getting toxins out of your food and your environment will help you to lose weight and stay healthy.

In her book *Toxic Overload,* Pamela Baillie-Hamilton suggests that instead of evaluating foods in terms of conventional calories, you should evaluate a food's chemical calorie content and its ability to damage your natural slimming system. "Lettuce, unless it is organic, is more fattening than an avocado because it contains far more chemical calories," she writes. "This is because it is a relatively fragile food crop that tends to be sprayed repeatedly, while the avocado is a much more robust crop that needs hardly any intervention at all."

So-called fattening chemicals can range from hormones and antibiotics fed to the animals that you consume, to the cleaning products you use on your carpet, or the artificial sweeteners in your diet drinks. To prevent and reverse disease and control your weight, you must limit exposure to toxins. We have no personal control over many of the chemicals in our environment, which is why we must be especially diligent about avoiding those toxins over which we do have control. Small toxic exposures each day from many sources such as breakfast cereal, toothpaste, shampoo, soap, perfume, deodorant, hair dye, newspapers, magazines, furnaces, hot water heaters, exhaust fumes, carpets, mattresses, dry cleaning, a new car, or a newly painted room can add up to toxic overload. When the amount of toxins coming in exceeds our capacity to detoxify them, the result is toxic overload and disease.

A Silent, Invisible, and Deadly Problem

Man-made chemicals can compel you to eat more than you need and to store fat instead of burning it. To prevent and reverse disease and achieve permanent weight control, it is essential to learn how to:

- Avoid exposure to toxins.
- Assist your body's detoxification systems.
- Lower your existing load of stored toxins.

Virtually every American is in toxic overload, which causes cells to malfunction, failing to properly communicate, self-regulate, and self-repair. These failures throw the body out of balance, creating disease. Toxins interfere with cell chemistry in a variety of ways. Toxins can disable critical enzymes or interfere with hormone activity. They can signal genes to "turn on" inappropriately. Toxins can interfere with the light and electrical signals that control intercellular communications, and also limit the distance these signals can travel, even stopping signals from reaching their destination. This causes chaos in the body's communications and feedback systems, resulting in disregulation and disease.

Virtually all the air we breathe, the food we eat, the water we drink, the soil in which we grow our food, the buildings we live and work in, and even the clothes we wear are contaminated with toxic, man-made chemicals. Toxins are so prevalent that avoiding all of them is impossible, and they are piling up too quickly for the body to get rid of them. The average person is now bioaccumulating (storing) between three hundred and five hundred industrial chemicals in his or her body. These chemicals can interfere with the body's natural detoxification systems and deplete our nutrient reserves at alarming rates. Some of these chemicals, such as flame retardants, have reached concentrations in humans that are known to cause disease in animals. Every year, American industry produces more than a million tons of toxic waste, and more than a billion pounds of herbicides, pesticides, and fungicides are dumped into our environment, contaminating our soil, air, food, and water. Most of our water supplies are contaminated with traces of hundreds of these toxins, and a number of them exceed existing safety guidelines. To make matters worse, toxins such as chlorine and fluoride are deliberately added to our water.

We use personal-care products such as toothpaste and shampoo that are loaded with toxins that go right through our mucus membranes and skin. Modern medicine adds to the problem by prescribing medications made of toxic chemicals that suppress the symptoms of disease but do not treat its true causes. Half the population is on these toxic drugs, and to make matters worse, these chemicals are now contaminating our drinking water supplies. We are exposed to more toxins, and in far greater concentrations, than anyone before in history. The result is toxic overload, disease, and overweight.

These man-made chemicals introduce molecules that the body has never been exposed to before and is inadequately prepared to detoxify. The number and variety of toxins accumulating in our bodies compounds the problem. We now understand that these chemicals, even in minute concentrations, when acting in combination, can be thousands of times more toxic than when acting alone.

If You Look for Fat-Free, Look for Toxin-Free

Toxic food additives can damage your weight-control systems and cause weight gain, even if you cut down on calories. A client named Anthony discovered this after trying fifteen years of diets and weight-loss schemes that had failed to produce permanent results. Anthony's doctor suggested his weight problem might be genetic. On his own, Anthony had actually improved his eating habits (cutting out most sugar and adding in more fresh food and exercise), but he continued to drink diet colas daily, exposing him to aspartame, and to eat out regularly at a favorite Chinese restaurant, exposing him to monosodium glutamate (MSG). In addition, he frequently consumed processed foods, which left him open to a host of other chemical additives. Once Anthony, at five foot ten, got toxins out of his life, he dropped from 242 pounds to 170, which is what can happen when the toxins are no longer jamming your appetite and fat-burning controls. Artificial sweeteners such as aspartame and flavor enhancers such as MSG are common culprits in increasing weight, and many people consume these every day.

Among the other toxic weight-enhancers ingested with food are pesticides such as carbamates and organophosphates.

Other weight-enhancers include organochlorines, PCBs, solvents, heavy metals, and chemicals leached from plastics such
as phthalates and bisphenol A. Growth promoters such as
steroids, antibiotics, and pesticides are fed to animals to make
them fatten up faster on less food, but they have the same
effect on people who eat the meat from these animals. Steroids
fed to cattle make them gain 20 percent more weight on 15
percent less food. More than 70 percent of the antibiotics used
in America are used for the purpose of fattening animals
(as well as keeping them free of infections), causing chickens,
pigs, and cows to gain up to 8 percent in weight. Organophosphate pesticides have been used to fatten livestock. This
is no longer permitted, but it still happens. Unfortunately,
organophosphates are still commonly used on fruits and vegetables. Carbamates are another widely used class of pesticide
that has a powerful effect on weight gain in animals.
Carbamates are also found in high levels on potatoes, peanuts,
citrus fruits, and other fruits and vegetables. Organochlorines
such as PCBs, DDT, and lindane are also powerful growth
promoters and weight enhancers. Although now banned in the
United States, they remain in the environment, and farm animals continue to ingest them. Most farmed salmon are highly
contaminated with PCBs. Bisphenol A is a component of
polycarbonate plastics, a material used to make many consumer items, including baby bottles and large water bottles.
This chemical has been found to induce insulin resistance,
which contributes to overweight, at doses five thousand times
below the dose identified by the EPA as causing effects. Most
of these chemicals are fat soluble, and as our bodies are not
designed to get rid of fat-soluble chemicals, they are stored in
our fatty tissues and remain there for decades, continuing to
cause us harm, including weight gain.

Toxins stored in our fatty tissues harm us in numerous
ways. One way is by disabling fat-processing enzymes in fat
cells, causing the fat to stay where it is. Another is by poison-

ing fat-burning enzymes in muscle cells, depriving those cells of energy and causing loss of muscle tissue and fat-burning capacity. The down-regulation and disabling of fat-burning enzymes is an important factor in overweight disease.

Paula Baillie-Hamilton had this to say about the effects of toxins on weight-controlling hormones:

> Virtually every chemical found in our food appears to have a significant effect on at least one of the major weight-controlling hormones. More specifically, these chemicals tended to increase the levels of fattening hormones such as insulin and steroids, while reducing the levels of slimming hormones such as thyroid, sex and growth hormones and catecholamines. . . . Catecholamines control our appetite and "set" our energy levels and our desire to exercise. Any fall in their levels will not only reduce the amount of voluntary exercise we feel like taking, but will also probably lessen the involuntary movements that we don't even notice. Synthetic chemicals can interfere with the way that our bodies absorb nutrients from foods, destroy some of the more delicate nutrients, prevent the production of other essential nutrients and even increase the rate at which the body excretes nutrients.

Heavy metals such as mercury, lead, and cadmium have been linked to obesity, even at low levels that were previously thought to be safe. According to a study at the Harvard School of Public Health reported in the October 21, 1995, issue of *Science News,* children with the highest bone levels of lead gained the most weight and were 50 percent more likely to suffer from high blood pressure.

We have already discussed the ways in which common flavor enhancers such as MSG cause weight gain. Enhancing flavor is especially important to the processed food industry because food loses flavor, as well as nutrients, during processing. MSG and other flavor enhancers are added in order to make poor-quality food taste good, or at least to trick your brain into thinking, "Wow! This is great. I want more." Flavor enhancers, however, are excitotoxins, which have a devastating toxic effect on the body, damaging and destroying brain cells and causing weight gain.

Virtually all processed foods in jars, cans, and packages contain MSG and other food additives in one form or another, which interfere with your efforts to lose weight. The fact that MSG causes overweight has been known for decades. In 1969, researcher John Olney discovered that MSG caused obesity in experimental animals, and since then other researchers have demonstrated this same effect. In fact, exposure to MSG early in life can damage your weight-control systems for a lifetime. MSG damages a part of the brain (part of the hypothalamus) that inhibits appetite and promotes fat burning. MSG also stimulates the production of excess insulin, which we know has a number of serious negative effects, including inhibiting fat burning and increasing sugar cravings. The brain damage caused by MSG also inhibits the action of the hormone leptin, which is needed to control appetite and fat storage. Most overweight people have high levels of leptin in their bloodstream, but it isn't working for them because their brain receptors have been damaged.

MSG is disguised on food labels in words such as *natural flavors, spices, hydrolyzed vegetable protein, vegetable protein, sodium caseinate, textured protein, soy protein extract,* and others. All of these contain glutamate, the biologically active part of monosodium glutamate. Even baby formula can contain glutamate in the form of caseinate. When you start to look for it, you may be shocked at how often you will find glutamate—it's everywhere. Dr. Russell Blaylock observed in his book *Health and Nutrition Secrets,* "One of the worst offenders is pizza, especially commercial pizza. The tomato sauce is high in naturally derived free glutamate alone. When you add to this a liberal helping of MSG additive, you have a very neurotoxic mix."

Adding to Dr. Blaylock's comment on neurotoxicity is a January 2006 study reported in *Toxicological Sciences*. Researchers at the University of Liverpool found that when MSG was combined with a blue food coloring, nerve cells stopped growing and nerve signaling was impaired. Further, the effect of both acting together was four times greater than either acting alone. A similar experiment was performed with aspartame and a yellow food coloring. The combined effect on nerve cells was seven times greater than each alone. In the experiments, these additives were combined in the same concentrations that reflect a typical children's snack drink; then we wonder why our children are overweight and having problems in school. Remember, food additives are licensed one at a time and are almost never tested in combination. Unfortunately, we and our children are consuming such combinations of toxins every day in processed foods. Every time you buy a processed food, whether it be smoked fish, pasta sauce, a jar of pickles, processed cheese, a dessert, breakfast cereal, candy, or prepared meals, unless you know a lot of chemistry, you have no idea what you are buying. Worse, you have no idea what it is doing to your body.

Remember, too, that the labels do not list toxic chemical residues, such as the mercury in tuna or the pesticides and hormones contained in meat and dairy. Artificial ripening agents are often used on fruits and vegetables that have been harvested before ripening in order to be transported long distances for sale. Bananas, for example, are picked green and usually treated with ethylene gas to cause them to ripen faster once they have reached their destination, which is why organic bananas ripen more slowly than their conventional counterparts.

The Deception of Diet Sodas

The artificial sweetener aspartame is used in diet drinks and foods and marketed as a way to replace sugar and control weight. In truth, aspartame does affect weight—it makes you fat! Aspartate, a component of aspartame, has the same ability as glutamate to destroy brain cells. Like MSG, aspartame also damages the part of the brain that is sensitive to the appetite-suppressing and fat-burning control of leptin. Like MSG, aspartame stimulates insulin production, thus inhibiting fat burning and creating sugar cravings.

Dr. Blaylock addressed aspartame in *The Blaylock Wellness Letter:* "Unbelievably, dietitians, medical doctors and many public institutions are promoting the use of 'diet' soft drinks and other food sweetened with aspartame (NutraSweet®, Equal®, etc.) as the answer to the problems of obesity." That aspartame promotes obesity has been proven in numerous studies, including a 1997 study published in the *International Journal of Obesity* where it was determined that people ate significantly more food when they drank aspartame-sweetened beverages. Yet, an estimated 70 percent of the U.S. population uses aspartame, including 40 percent of our children. It is a deadly neurotoxin that also can cause diabetes, aggravate diabetic retinopathy and neuropathy, destroy the optic nerve, keep blood sugar out of control, and cause diabetics to go into convulsions. It is also known to contribute to cancer and Alzheimer's disease.

Other Toxins to Avoid

While the preceding toxins have the greatest effect on weight control, keep in mind that all toxins, to at least some degree, not only damage your health but can affect your weight. Following is a list of other sources of toxins to be minimized or avoided.

Natural Toxins

Foods can be contaminated with "natural" toxins produced by bacteria and molds, often invisible to the consumer. Toxins produced by molds are called mycotoxins. Certain foods such as corn, peanuts, grapes, raisins, other dried fruits, beer, cheeses, fermented foods, bottled fruit juices, and berries that are not farm fresh are more likely to be moldy than others. Aflatoxin is a particularly dangerous mycotoxin. It is found on figs, grains, nuts, and seeds, and especially peanuts (including peanut butter), pistachios, walnuts, and corn (including items such as corn syrup, corn starch, corn meal, corn flakes, corn chips, and corn tortillas). Grains should be purchased as fresh as possible, or they may be too moldy and toxic.

Toxin-producing bacteria can be present in almost any food when it is purchased. Fresh fruits and vegetables can be washed to eliminate most bacteria. Always smell meat, fish, and poultry before cooking or eating. Commercial milk products are contaminated with bacteria, often far in excess of government guidelines.

Toxins from Food Packaging

Toxins in packaging materials such as plastic wrap, plastic bottles, canned foods and drinks, milk containers, juice boxes, and Styrofoam can leach polymers, plasticizers, stabilizers, fillers, and even colorants into our food. Styrene found in Styrofoam drinking cups and food packaging is now found in 100 percent of human tissue in America.

Cooking Up Toxins

Toxins are produced when food is cooked. The best choice is slow cooking at low temperatures. The worst choices for food preparation are barbecuing and microwaving.

When food is heated above 375 degrees (as in toasting, frying, grilling, broiling, and even baking), toxic compounds, which are powerful carcinogens, are produced. The higher the cooking temperature and the longer the cooking time, the more toxins are formed. Blackened foods are absolutely not acceptable.

Microwaving food is a dreadful choice. Research at the Swiss Federal Institute of Technology in 1992 found that volunteers who ate microwaved food experienced decreased blood hemoglobin and increased white cell counts—lowering the amount of vital oxygen available to cells and stressing the immune system. The nutritional quality of microwaved food is decreased 60 to 90 percent. A November 2003 study published in the *Journal of the Science of Food and Agriculture* reported that microwaved broccoli lost 97 percent of its antioxidants; only 11 percent were lost when steamed.

Pots and Pans Could Be Trouble

After making healthy food choices and selecting high-quality ingredients, it would be a shame to add toxins to your foods with the wrong cookware. The best pots and pans are those made of glass, stoneware, ceramic-coated metal, or ceramics such as CorningWare. Other materials interact with food and introduce toxins. If you must use something other than the safest choices, choose stainless steel. The worst choices are aluminum and pans with Teflon coatings.

Genetically Modified Foods

Eating genetically modified organism (GMO) foods presents risks with unknown dimensions. Studies have demonstrated serious health effects when GMO foods are fed to laboratory animals, yet 75 percent of the foods sold in U.S. supermarkets contain GMOs. Genetically modified foods are unnatural, and no one has any idea of their future health consequences. Inserting foreign genes into genetic material is not a precise process; it is all too easy to obtain unintended results that lower nutritional content, create harmful allergens, or generate unique toxins. The effects of these changes may not become known for years. The best way to avoid GMOs is to eat organically produced food. Even then, organically produced soy and corn are now contaminated with the GMO variety.

Polluted Water

Water is essential for life and effective weight control, but water is also a source of toxins. These toxins can deactivate critical enzymes and create hormonal imbalances that affect your appetite and weight-control systems, as well as cause cancer. The EPA has cited 129 chemicals in tap water as serious health risks. Most tap water in this country is not healthy to drink or even to use for showers or baths.

Chlorine is a toxin deliberately added to our water supply. Chlorine kills harmful microorganisms, but it also damages health. Consuming chlorinated water increases the risk for birth defects and miscarriages, as well as for a variety of cancers, and also kills good bacteria in our intestinal tract. Some researchers believe that bathing and swimming in chlorinated water is contributing to the skin cancer epidemic. Chlorine reacts with organic matter present in the water, producing a family of chemicals called trihalomethanes, which are carcinogenic even in minute amounts.

Fluoride, another toxin deliberately added to water, does little or nothing to prevent tooth decay, while it damages health. Fluoride is a powerful enzyme poison. It disrupts thyroid enzymes, suppressing thyroid function and causing weight gain. Children can be more susceptible to obesity if their mothers drank fluoridated water while pregnant, resulting in partial underactivity of the thyroid in the child. Fluoride damages teeth, bones, kidneys, muscles, nerves, and the brain, and also causes cancer, osteoporosis, and suppressed immunity.

Ninety million Americans are consuming tap water contaminated with arsenic, a powerful human carcinogen. In addition, arsenic damages the digestive, cardiovascular, neurological, reproductive, and immune systems. Arsenic is a contaminant in the toxic industrial-waste product used to fluoridate most of our water.

Fifty million Americans drink aluminum-contaminated water. An aluminum salt (alum) is added to water to "clarify" it by helping to settle and remove particulate and organic matter. This process leaves aluminum residue in the water. While we are actually exposed to more aluminum in our food, the aluminum in water is far more bioavailable, making it a more troublesome source. Aluminum is a neurotoxin and has been associated with Alzheimer's disease, Parkinson's disease, and ALS (amyotrophic lateral sclerosis), commonly called Lou Gehrig's disease.

Tap water that is contaminated with nitrates and nitrites is available to 100 million Americans, especially in agricultural areas from fertilizer runoff and animal waste. Nitrates are readily converted to nitrites by microorganisms. Nitrites are especially dangerous for infants and sick people because they decrease the ability of hemoglobin to carry oxygen, and they form powerful carcinogens called nitrosamines.

Given the problems with most tap water, protecting ourselves is essential. The most practical and economical solution for pure drinking water is to use a high-quality reverse-osmosis system (see appendix D for recommendations). Use a filter on your shower. Beware, too, of breathing the fumes from dishwashers and washing machines because of toxic bleaches and detergents.

Beware Breathing the Indoor Air

Many of the chemicals we breathe have the potential to affect our appetite, fat storage controls, and weight. The most polluted air we breathe can be found right in our own homes or offices. Indoor air is typically two to five times more polluted than outdoor air, and can easily reach a hundred times greater pollution. Because most Americans spend 90 percent of their time indoors, this is a significant hazard. Fortunately, we can control the quality of this air by minimizing the number of toxins we introduce as well as using air filters to reduce our exposure.

Indoor pollution comes from sources such as building materials, furnishings, gas appliances, air conditioning and heating systems, cleaning and consumer products, tobacco smoke, and carpets. Synthetic-fiber carpets are a major source of indoor pollution. As many as two hundred chemicals come out of the fibers, adhesives, backing, and padding, causing irregular heartbeat, fatigue, rashes, memory loss, muscle pain, blurred vision, and tremors. Mice exposed to fumes from new carpets die in a matter of hours, and even carpets up to twelve years old can cause severe neurological problems. If these fumes can kill mice, what are they doing to you, your children, and your pets? Use carpets made of natural fiber or hardwood floors with natural-fiber area rugs.

Carpet-cleaning products contain a multitude of toxic ingredients, making matters worse. Carpet shampoos leave a residue on carpet fibers, and those residues can disperse into the air or be picked up by pets and children who are close to the carpet. Carpet cleaning leaves carpets wet for too long, encouraging the growth of mold. Even when mold is not actively growing, mold particles and spores can cause health problems, such as fatigue, headaches, allergy symptoms, and asthma attacks. Chemicals from molds can mimic hormones as well as cause cancer (see Appendix D for safe carpet-cleaning recommendations).

Dangerous gases and particles also are generated by household appliances such as gas stoves, water heaters, furnaces, space heaters, and fireplaces, which can release toxins such as nitrogen dioxide, carbon monoxide, methane, and other gasses along with fine particles. Furnaces and gas water heaters should be kept outside the living space, such as in a shed or unattached garage. If this is not possible, consider switching to an electric water heater. Gas stoves should be used only with good ventilation; an electric stove is preferable. Never use artificial logs in the fireplace as they release a heavy hydrocarbon load into the living space.

Other chemicals contributing to indoor air pollution include paradichlorobenzene, found in mothballs and deodorizers; exhaust fumes and hydrocarbon vapors coming from cars in attached garages; pesticides used in or around the home (known to affect weight control); tobacco smoke, perfume, cosmetics, cleaning products, aerosol products, and all manner of products scented with synthetic fragrances.

Dry-cleaned clothing has an odor from toxic solvent residues. Air out such clothing by hanging it in the garage until the smell is gone, or pick it up a week after it is ready, allowing it time to release the toxins.

Personal-Care Products Cause Harm

Most personal-care products—such as makeup, deodorant, and moisturizers—include toxins that will not only make you feel worse, but also look older. Most of the products available in department stores, drugstores, supermarkets, and even expensive boutiques contain toxic chemicals in the form of fragrances, coloring agents, moisturizers, foaming agents, and preservatives. Even most of the choices at health-food stores contain harmful toxins. Our rule is: *if a product cannot be ingested without harming you, then it is not safe enough to put on your skin, hair, nails, or teeth.*

Many of the chemicals contained in personal-care products are easily absorbed through the skin or mucous membranes. Especially dangerous are those products such as sunscreen, lotions, and makeup that are left on the skin for long periods of time. These usually contain preservatives known to damage and age skin. Most commercial toothpaste comes with a warning on the label about not swallowing or ingesting it due to its toxicity. However, even when it is not swallowed, fluoride and other toxins in toothpaste can enter your bloodstream through the permeable membranes in your mouth.

Antibacterial soaps and creams are another source of toxins. Most antibacterial products contain triclosan, which is absorbed through the skin. Triclosan is designed to kill bacteria (cells) and is now showing up in alarming amounts in human breast milk.

Fragrances in soaps, lotions, kitty litter, cleaners, and perfumes are toxic. Although fragrances were originally made from flowers and herbs, today most fragrances are made of toxic synthetic petrochemicals, which are not only carcinogenic, but neurotoxic, poisoning the nervous system. Manufacturers of these products are not required to list ingredients on their labels.

Deodorants are another class of toxic products. Most deodorants (even deodorant stones, which are touted as healthy) contain aluminum, a suspected contributor to Alzheimer's disease, chemical sensitivities, and breast cancer. Aluminum-free deodorants often contain toxic triclosan. See Appendix D for a safe recommendation.

Many women treat their face daily with potions designed to make them look better. Unfortunately, most of these products contain chemicals that are known to age skin, making them look worse. For example, parabens, which are used as preservatives, will damage sublayers of the skin worse than severe sunburn. From personal-care items alone, the average woman might be exposed to one hundred toxic chemicals a day.

Following is a partial list of the toxins to avoid in your personal-care products. Recall that toxins can be thousands of times more toxic when acting together. You should also carry this list with you when you go to the store.

aluminum compounds
artificial fragrances
benzaldehyde (shaving foams)
benzyl acetate (aftershave)
BHA
BHT
butylenes glycol (hair spray)
colors
cresol
DEA
detergents
EDTA
ethyl acetate (aftershave)
flavors
fluoride
formaldehyde
glycols
ketoconazole (antifungal)
nickel sulfate
nitrates

octylmethoxycinnamate
  (sunscreens)
parabens (a class of preservatives ending with paraben)
phenol
phthalates (moisturizers, nail
  polish)
potassium bromate (toothpaste)
quaternium-15 (shampoos)
resorcinol
selenium sulfide
sodium cetyl sulfate
sodium laureth sulfate
sodium lauryl sulfate
TEA
trichloroethylene
triclosan (antibacterial)
violet 2 or 4B
zinc pyrithione (dandruff
  shampoo)

Unhealthy Cleaning

Household products can actually make your house "dirty" because they add toxins to your living space. Almost all commercial cleaning products and air fresheners are toxic. No chemical should ever come in contact with your skin unless you know it is safe. Dangerous solvents in cleaners and household products can injure your kidneys and liver. Some common toxic household chemicals include ammonia, chlorine bleach, aerosol propellants, detergents, petroleum distillates, and toluene. If you cannot avoid using a toxic cleaner, wear gloves and keep the area well ventilated. Do not breathe aerosol or spray products.

Laundry rooms are also toxic sites. Detergents, bleach, spot removers, and fabric softeners all contain toxins. Replace synthetic detergents with natural soap-based products. Chlorine bleach can be replaced with safer oxygen bleaches, sodium percarbonate, or hydrogen peroxide. Seventh Generation brand products are acceptable alternatives for laundry use.

Pesticides

Most insecticides are neurotoxic to insects. Unfortunately, they also damage your own nervous system and make you fat. Insecticides can have estrogen-like effects that lead to cancer, birth defects, and fertility problems. They have also been linked to Parkinson's disease and numerous other medical problems. For a recommendation on a safe insecticide, see Appendix D. One way to avoid pesticides is to eat organically grown foods.

A Prescription for Poor Health

Prescription drugs are another source of toxins that contribute to overweight by interfering with appetite and fat storage controls. It is known that antipsychotics, antidepressants, and other prescription drugs such as steroids can cause patients to gain weight. People who gain weight on drugs often report feeling hungrier and developing intense cravings for sugar and high-carbohydrate foods. Prescription drugs are just one more reason that people have difficulty losing weight, and it should not be a surprise that overweight has become epidemic along with the explosive growth of prescription drugs.

In fact, the official information sheets for many of the most frequently prescribed drugs list weight gain as a side effect. Further, these drugs can be insidious in that it may take years for the weight gain to become apparent, and weight gain may continue even a year after treatment ends. Tens of millions of people are taking such drugs to control their depression, blood pressure, cholesterol, diabetes, heartburn, and inflammation, as well as drugs used to treat mental disorders such as bipolar disorder and schizophrenia. Hormone replacement therapy and oral contraceptives containing estrogen can cause increased appetite as well as fluid retention. Even over-the-counter drugs are known to affect weight. For example, the antihistamine diphenhydramine can cause weight gain and is listed as an ingredient in numerous sleep aids as well as cold and allergy preparations.

As you are aware by now, insulin causes weight gain. Prior to the 1990s, diabetics took one insulin shot per day. Now they take multiple shots to do a better job of controlling their disease. However, diabetics on this "intensive therapy" gain an average of ten pounds more than those taking one shot per day.

Are we recommending that you quit taking all of your prescription drugs right now? Absolutely not. We are recommending that you consider why you came to need the drugs in the first place. We urge you to seek safer alternatives and find a physician and other professionals who will work with you to help you to address the true causes of your ailments and to get you off the drugs. Your body was designed to be self-healing. Giving it toxic drugs will defeat your goals of normal weight and optimal health.

Send Those Toxins on Their Way

Your body produces a substantial toxic load every day as a result of normal metabolism. Very simply, all your cell factories produce industrial waste as they produce the life-giving chemicals you need to function. To cope with this, as well as with toxins coming in from the outside, the body is equipped with a complex detoxification system. Various organs in the body—the liver, kidneys, bowels, lungs, lymph system, and the skin—are part of that complex system. Water promotes detoxification through the kidneys and sweat glands. Sweating assists in the removal of water-soluble toxins. Fiber helps "carry out the garbage" in the digestive system, and exercise also helps us detoxify by initiating sweating and encouraging the movement of toxins through the lymphatic system.

Your job is to help your detoxification system work by providing adequate nutrients and to reduce your exposure to toxins, preventing system overload. Supporting the liver is especially important. At any given time, about 25 percent of all the blood in your body is in your liver—to be detoxified. Enzymes, produced by the liver, deactivate and eliminate toxins. Interfering with these enzymes by introducing environmental toxins such as lead and mercury, or never manufacturing them because of nutrient deficiency, results in toxic overload.

Detoxification by the liver occurs in two phases: In phase I, the liver produces enzymes that take harmful toxins such as alcohol, prescription drugs, pesticides, and herbicides and oxidizes them (burns them) in preparation for removal from the body. This process creates potentially harmful free radicals that must be neutralized with dietary antioxidant nutrients.

In phase II, more enzymes are used to combine the oxidized chemicals from phase I with other molecules, and the combination can then be excreted harmlessly in the bile or urine. In both phases, the food we eat supplies the raw materials needed to produce all of the necessary enzymes and other chemicals required. Our amazing detoxification systems depend on a constant supply of nutrients, which we must get from our diet, but frequently do not.

Help your liver's phase I detoxification process with these nutrients: vitamins A, C, and E, along with coenzyme Q_{10}, carotenoids, bioflavonoids, selenium, manganese, copper, and zinc. Some of the above neutralize free radicals directly—others activate enzymes that neutralize them. Red, yellow, purple, orange, and green vegetables are loaded with antioxidant nutrients needed for detoxification.

Assist phase II detoxification with cruciferous vegetables, such as cabbage, broccoli, cauliflower, garlic, onions, leeks, kale, and Brussels sprouts. These vegetables enable the liver to eliminate powerful carcinogens, helping to protect us from cancer. Supplements, including reduced glutathione, alpha lipoic acid, N-acetylcysteine, and glutamine, are all helpful. These dietary suggestions combined with high-quality supplements keep your liver's toxic defenses at peak function.

Much of your body is made of water; the kidneys need it to excrete water-soluble toxins. Water constantly moves throughout your body and must be changed frequently to keep your system healthy. As a rule of thumb, about eight glasses of pure water should be consumed every day. Your water supply must be pure, so as not to add to your toxic load. Water should be consumed as water alone, not in beverages such as coffee, tea, or alcohol (these substances actually cause the body to lose water). Water is often overlooked; therefore, dehydration is a common problem—especially among the elderly.

Lose Toxins and Burn Calories in a Sauna

Avoiding new toxins and supporting your detoxification system are essential, but not the whole answer to toxic overload. You must also rid your body of toxins that have already accumulated. Most likely decades worth of health-damaging toxins are in your tissues, putting constant stress on your body. This accumulation gets in the way of efforts to lose or keep off unwanted weight. It is very important that this load be reduced and not allowed to reaccumulate. As you make changes and begin to incorporate the *NBFA* Lifestyle, we strongly encourage regular use of a sauna as the only reliable way to get rid of accumulated oil-soluble toxins.

Our bodies were designed before the petroleum age began, which happened only a century ago. Since then, our environment has become a sea of oil-soluble toxins. Never before exposed to such toxins, our bodies are not designed to get rid of them. As a result, the average person is bioaccumulating hundreds of man-made chemicals, from the styrene found in disposable cups to PCBs, dioxins, paradichlorobenzene (in mothballs and deodorizers), sodium lauryl sulfate (in soap, shampoo, and toothpaste), formaldehyde (plywood, particle-board, and permanent-press clothing), triclosan (in antibacterial soap and underarm deodorants), and many others. Fire retardants (from carpets, mattresses, cars, upholstered furniture, TVs, and computers) are now being found in alarming quantities in human tissue and breast milk. Man-made, fat-promoting pesticides such as organophosphates, organochlorines, and carbamates can be stored for decades in your tissues from past exposures, even if you are now eating organic foods. If these chemicals are jamming your fat-control mechanisms, it will be very difficult to lose weight until you lose the chemicals.

Heat causes cells to release toxins, and hyperthermic (sweat) treatments have been used for health purposes by cultures around the world for millennia. American Indians, for example, used sweat lodges. Hyperthermic practices are known to reduce levels of organic toxins such as pesticides and PCBs, as well as heavy metals such as lead and mercury.

The skin is the body's largest organ and an important part of the body's detoxification system. Saunas melt the fat layer in the skin, allowing the oil to ooze out of the oil glands along with its cargo of accumulated fat-soluble toxins. In addition, water-soluble toxins such as heavy metals are lost in the sweat. Over time, it is possible to reduce one's toxic load substantially and to keep it low.

Saunas are better than a steam room or wet heat because the body temperature can be kept lower, which enables you to remain in the sauna longer. The oils need more time to ooze out onto the skin. After a sauna, it is critical to wash off with pure castile soap, such as Dr. Bronner's. This washes away the toxins so they don't get reabsorbed into the skin. It is also important to stay well hydrated while using the sauna.

Saunas are available at gyms and health clubs. If you use a commercial sauna, lie prone on the lowest bench. This will expose your body to a manageable temperature, allowing you to spend more time. We recommend starting slowly and gradually working your way up to an hour or more. You also can use your time in the sauna to do other healthy things such as eye exercises or meditation.

Infrared saunas are easier for most people to use because the air temperature in that type of sauna can be kept much lower, while still being effective. In fact, infrared saunas are even more effective at detoxifying than traditional electrically heated saunas. Most of the saunas available for purchase or health-club use are made of woods, as well as solvent-based adhesives, sealants, and lacquers, that give off toxic chemicals. Since the purpose of the sauna is to get rid of toxic chemicals, sitting in a toxic sauna is counterproductive (see Appendix D for recommendations about nontoxic saunas).

Far-infrared, invisible wavelengths of the infrared spectrum, has been extensively studied and found to have numerous health benefits. Far-infrared has the same effect as the warming rays of the sun, and easily penetrates human tissue, creating a natural resonance with water molecules, providing many beneficial effects. Infrared saunas require less electricity than conventional hot-rock saunas. They are more economical, heat up faster, and usually run on ordinary house current.

Many people do not like saunas, and many with health problems cannot tolerate them. Their experience with conventional saunas is that the excessively hot air is too harsh and uncomfortable. Even under these harsh conditions, the heat penetration from conventional saunas is superficial, penetrating only a few millimeters. Far-infrared saunas are a different experience. The infrared heats you rather than the air so the penetration is more than one and a half inches deep. This is desirable for healing tissue and releasing toxins. Meanwhile, the air temperature is kept at a comfortable and controllable level—100–120°F versus 130–180°F in a conventional sauna.

With almost every American in toxic overload, regular sauna use is a necessity for those who care about their health and who want to maintain a healthy weight. Studies show that a combination of daily exercise, nutrition through diet and supplements, along with regular saunas provides powerful benefits. Sherry Rogers, author of *Detoxify or Die,* has called saunas both a "household necessity" and a "weekly necessity forever."

Saunas help you lose weight in another way as well. An infrared sauna can burn up to six hundred calories in thirty minutes, without you moving a muscle. A sauna session can be the calorie-burning equivalent of rowing a boat for thirty minutes or running several miles. In fact, a far-infrared sauna is the only natural, healthy way to burn calories without exercise. Many people who have tried to lose weight by dieting alone have been pleasantly surprised by the results of using an infrared sauna. If you can afford it, put one in your home. For those who cannot afford it or do not have space for a sauna, regular visits to a health club or sauna facility are a must.

THE MENTAL 7 PATHWAY

Thinking Yourself Thin

Your thoughts can have a powerful effect on your health and weight. Some things you'll learn in this chapter are:

- How to transform your thinking so that it is an asset to your weight loss rather than a hindrance.
- How to create a vision of health that you desire to achieve.
- How to set specific, realistic, and measurable goals.
- How to identify emotional eating and create strategies to overcome it.
- Prayer and meditation can be powerful tools in your quest.
- Lightening up and laughing can improve your health.

The first place we must win the victory is in our own minds.
If you don't think you can be successful, then you never will
be. If you don't think your body can be healed, it never will be.

—Joel Osteen
Your Best Life Now

You are what you eat, but you also are what you think. You
can truly think yourself thinner and healthier as readily as you
can mentally sabotage your health and weight loss.

The mind and body are inseparable. To look and feel years
younger and be pounds thinner, the process begins in your
mind. Food is powerfully connected with your emotions.
Many of the reasons people eat—and, too often, overeat—
have nothing to do with hunger, but instead with their feelings,
habits, and addictions, which is a major reason that many
people cannot lose weight or keep off the weight they lose.

What you conjure up in your mind is as important as what
you prepare to eat. The Mental Pathway can lead you toward
powerful ways of thinking and believing that help to prevent
disease, renew vitality, and lose weight permanently. Few of us
recognize the power of our own minds. Even fewer know how
to effectively use that power. Learning how to visualize a slim
new you, set reachable goals, and affirm your vision—out
loud, especially—are critical steps toward weight-loss success.

Believe, in Order to Achieve

The activity of our mind affects every cell in our body. The
reason that placebos work is that what we believe largely
determines what we achieve. The body is an obedient servant.
It does what you tell it to do. The body is listening every
moment of the day, and we are all constantly giving it instructions, whether we are aware of it or not. Unfortunately, all too

often those instructions are negative ones that only add to our problems. If you keep telling your body it is fat or sick, it will obediently comply and keep you that way. This makes it difficult to get well or lose weight. How much better it would be if you were, several times every day, to tell your body it is healthy and trim—right now! It eventually gets the message and follows your instructions.

We can use the incredible power of our brain to great benefit or waste, keeping us accomplished or defeated, youthful or debilitated, healthy or struggling with disease—including the disease of overweight. In too many ways and on too many days, we think small and we limit ourselves to mundane lives, making ourselves vulnerable to disease. Break out of this self-imposed mind-set, and you can harness the power of your thoughts and your beliefs in order to make radical changes in every realm of your life, including health and weight loss.

The Power of the Placebo

In his book *Peace, Love and Healing,* Dr. Bernie Siegel tells numerous stories that illustrate the power of the mind to control the body's health. One amazing success involved a young boy struggling with the ravages of a brain tumor, and his parents, who used the power of thinking and believing to ease their son's suffering and help restore his health.

> The parents used words to create positive expectations in the boy which were strong enough to diminish the side effects of some very powerful anticancer drugs. . . . The first time he took his CCNV [antinausea] pill we also gave him the recommended anti-emetic to lessen the nausea. He got very sick that night and was on the couch all the next day. The next time we gave it to him we told him that you only get sick the first time. . . . He said he felt much better this time and was up and about all the next day.

The same patient lost his hair due to the cancer treatment, and a placebo worked powerfully again. "To restore his hair growth we rubbed a 'magic mixture' on his head and told him it would make his hair grow. It did! When we stopped using it, it quit growing, and started growing again when we resumed putting it on."

In 1955, Dr. Henry K. Beecher, the first to mention the "placebo effect," wrote "The Powerful Placebo," published in the *Journal of the American Medical Association.* Beecher concluded that about one-third of the people who receive medical treatment show improvement simply because they believe that the treatment they are using will work (recent research is showing that up to 75 percent is the result of the placebo effect, and the true number is probably higher yet). In *Love, Medicine and Miracles,* Siegel tells the story of a cancer patient who came back from the brink of death, from lethargy to vitality, with his cancerous tumors melting like snowballs after he received an injection of water that he believed was a powerful new anticancer drug. Make no mistake, belief is essential to success.

What image do you have of yourself? Perhaps it is time to do a mental inventory and reshape that image. *You will never rise above the way you visualize yourself.* Don't focus on your fat or your weaknesses, but on your strengths. Envision your potential. Positive change rarely just happens. It must be envisioned, planned for, and sought after. Three practical steps can help you to harness the great power of your mind in order to optimize your health and well-being: visualize, set goals, and then put your mind to work.

It's Your Vision: Make It Great

Sadly, most of us take more time to plan our shopping list than we do to plan ways to ensure a future that is free of disease, including overweight. Here is a suggestion: In the coming week, set aside five to ten minutes a day to sit quietly and think about what you want to achieve. Visualize yourself free of excess pounds, with toned muscles, smooth and glowing skin, full of energy—and a radiant smile. Picture your cells healthy and functioning together optimally. Envision your physical problems or discouragements replaced by vigor and accomplishment. Let your imagination go. Become empowered by a vision of this ideal you. Believe that it can become a reality. Periodically throughout the day conjure up this focused image. Cast off doubt and remind yourself that countless others have used the power of their visualizations to conquer their weaknesses and to transform their lives.

In an article titled "The Mind and Weight Balance," published on the Hippocrates Health Institute website (www. hippocratesinstitute.org), Bob Del Monteque, a naturopathic doctor, tells how he was shocked when he ran into a formerly obese friend who now looked beautiful, fit, and years younger than before. She had always been a positive person; she had just lost herself in food. She told him that she had been able to transform her body using an unusual approach: She cut out a picture of the healthy, firm body of a well-known celebrity and replaced the star's face with a photograph of her own face. She placed this image all around her home. She used her mental will, a plant-based whole-food diet, and regular exercise to become the hard-bodied youth she had never been. In eight months, she lost ninety-three pounds and became a body builder and aerobic enthusiast. She is an example of what each of us can create when our vision is focused.

Don't Wander: Set Realistic Goals

Your next step is to set specific, measurable, and realistic goals. Goals are essential to help you chart how well you are doing and how much progress you are making. If you fail to set and work toward goals, you wander aimlessly. Jack Canfield, Mark Victor Hansen, and Les Hewitt, the authors of *The Power of Focus,* talk about the importance of goals:

"Consider the alternative—just drifting along aimlessly, hoping that one day good fortune will fall into your lap with little or no effort on your part. Wake up! You've got more chance of finding a grain of sugar on a sandy beach."

As you set goals, we encourage you to use the designated page in your *NBFA* Lifestyle journal to articulate them. (The pages for assembling this journal can be found in Appendices B and C. Complete instructions on preparing and using this journal are given in chapter 8. There is a section in this journal for you to list goals.) Think in terms of both short-term and long-term goals. In order for your goals to be empowering and motivating, they should be specific, measurable, and realistic. Don't set vague goals such as "lose weight," "get healthy," "change my lifestyle," and "start exercising." Be specific. The more detailed your goals are, the more helpful they will be. Set a weight-loss goal of, say, thirty or fifty pounds. Better yet, further define the goal, for instance, to lose an average of two pounds a week or eight pounds a month (with the realistic objective of dropping fifty pounds in seven or eight months). This also allows for plateaus and accounts for the slowing of weight loss as you near your ideal weight. This kind of goal is both measurable and realistic. If three months pass and you have lost twenty-five pounds, you will able to see that you are on course.

List the specific ways you want to change your lifestyle, including daily plans for achieving them and methods you plan to use to accomplish each purpose. As you consider adding exercise into your life, be specific: What kinds of exercise? What time of day? Where? For how long? How many days each week? Remember to be realistic and devise a strategy for each goal. Be sure to include goals for each of the pathways described in this book, as all of the pathways are essential to your success. After you write each goal, reexamine your goal and see if you can make it even more specific so that progress will be easily measured. Continually remind yourself to be reasonable rather than set yourself up for discouragement by making your goals excessively optimistic or rigid. Your goals provide you with motivation and accountability, and writing them down makes them more powerful. Picture the desired result of each goal as you create it, and become invigorated by the anticipation. Take the time often to reread your goals, visualizing the changes ahead. Continually check on your progress. In this way, you pursue your dreams, rather than just passively hope they might happen someday.

If you want to make yourself even more accountable, you might consider sharing your goals with a few trusted individuals. Select positive, optimistic people who will be supportive during this process. Don't waste time on pessimists; they are unable to help you visualize your achievements or encourage your pursuit.

Listen to Yourself, and Say It Out Loud

Now that you have visualized your future and set specific, achievable goals, it is time for action. Your first step is to believe that *you can* attain your goals. Begin each day with positive mental images of how you are changing. Affirm your dreams out loud. As you begin your day, repeat aloud positive affirmations. We all use affirmations, but many times we may get up and say, "I feel lousy," or "I am so stupid." Stop yourself when you are voicing negative affirmations and train yourself to think and speak positively. Here are some guidelines:

- State affirmations positively. Instead of saying "I am not fat," say "I am lean and muscular." Rather than "I am not tired," try "I am full of energy."
- State affirmations in the present tense as if they are already accomplished. Rather than "I will be disease free," say "My cells function perfectly" or "I am healthy and strong."
- State affirmations in language that your brain can readily accept. Don't repeat flowery or artificial terminology or

scientific words you have read if they are foreign to your way of thinking and talking. Your affirmations should sound like something you would naturally say.

- Keep affirmations short, picture what you say, and believe what you say. Repeat over and over—*five times is a minimum.*
- Affirmations should be stated aloud and with enthusiasm. Say it like you mean it and believe it: *"Every day, in every way I am stronger and healthier!"* Each time you repeat, be more emphatic. Since emotion is powerful, thoughts with emotion attached seem to have a greater impact on your mind. Hearing affirmations voiced with enthusiasm helps you to reset your mind and is vital to wellness.
- Begin with morning and evening affirmations. When you wake up, repeat them aloud; when you go to bed, say them again. Voicing them at bedtime allows your subconscious to dwell on them while you sleep. When you are unable to affirm out loud, don't miss the opportunity and instead do your affirmations silently.

When you are in the middle of an activity, affirm its usefulness. During your workout, you can say, "As I lift these weights I tone and build my muscles." "I am lean and fit." "As I eat this nutrient-rich food, I am giving my body the raw materials it needs to build healthy cells that will result in radiant skin and a strong immune system." "As I choose to forego temptations, I am choosing happiness rather than regret for my future." When doubtful or negative thoughts ensue, don't allow them to stay, but replace them by speaking the opposite aloud. You may be uncomfortable with all this at first—embarrassed even—but give it a chance because you will see that it does work.

Don't Let Your Friends Derail Your Efforts

The people in our lives play a major role in our thinking and can help or hinder our progress. Surrounding yourself with positive and encouraging people can have a profound impact on you. You need accountability and support from those who believe in you and will inspire you to have confidence and stay on track. At the outset, think of one or two people who will support your efforts to adopt the *NBFA* Lifestyle. Sadly, this is not always easy. You may be amazed by how many people live in negativity. When you are tempted to throw in the towel, to indulge in foods that are harmful or to forsake exercise, have someone positive you can contact who will help you to make wise, reasoned, and informed choices rather than emotional ones.

Negative people who see mostly defeat and gloom, who seem to almost enjoy thinking the worst, will infect those with whom they come into contact. If you spend time with someone like this, it is necessary for you to find people to help you maintain enthusiasm and confidence. Talk with any naysayers in your life and gently ask them to keep their opinions to themselves if they cannot support you in this lifestyle change.

Your efforts to lose weight and stay healthy may also be sabotaged if your friends and family are themselves overweight and have poor eating habits (unless they are making changes with you). It is likely that what you enjoy doing together is eating unhealthy and fattening foods. Most social events and outings revolve around food—usually food that includes the toxic Big Four, which promote weight gain and disease. You don't have to avoid these people, but you must be sure that they will not expect you to indulge with them. Seek to surround yourself with people who enjoy activities and other people more than they do junk food.

Are You Allergic or Addicted?

As we described in chapter 5, most overweight people are addicted to food, which is a powerful emotional force in overweight disease. One reason weight-loss diets don't work is that they fail to address addictions, and most addicted people are totally unaware that they are addicted. Refer back to chapter 5 to remind yourself how "feel good" chemicals produced in the brain when eating simple carbohydrates such as refined grains and sugars, as well as the "feel good" chemicals produced as a result of allergic reactions to foods, affect your emotions and behavior regarding food. In most overweight people, both of these mechanisms are at work, causing an addiction to both refined carbohydrates and allergenic foods.

Avoid these addictive foods and allergens, which you first must identify. One way to do that is by fasting for six days on water and buffered vitamin C. This technique is safe, inexpensive, and remarkably useful, but best to do under a practitioner's supervision. Reintroduce foods one at a time, recording how you feel—your emotions and your behaviors. You are most likely allergic to any food that causes you to feel tired, hot or flushed, have itchy eyes, runny nose, swollen fingers, puffy eyes, a bloated stomach, or skin eruptions.

Are You Eating Because You Are Hungry?

There are countless reasons for eating, and most of them have nothing to do with hunger. Food is, too often, an emotional crutch that we rely on to deal with trauma, loss, poor relationships, illness, fatigue, and other struggles. In order to successfully change your lifestyle, you need strategies to help you recognize and stop emotional eating behaviors. You cannot continue to seek solace in food and stay healthy and trim.

Emotional eating, also known as compulsive eating, is eating for reasons other than hunger. It is a major reason that many people can't lose weight and keep it off. We are all pro-grammed from infancy for emotional eating. When we cried, we were fed, but many times the cry was a cry of loneliness, discomfort, insecurity, boredom, sleepiness, anger, or something else. Since food was supplied as the solution no matter what the need, emotional eating became a learned behavior. Since we were comforted with food, we still turn to food for comfort when we are bored, angry, tired, lonely, stressed, or taxed in any way.

The best way to recognize emotional eating is by utilizing the *NBFA* Lifestyle journal. Accurately record *everything* you eat, and you will begin to notice when you eat for reasons other than hunger. As you record what you have eaten, ask yourself if you were hungry when you ate. Each time you eat when you are not hungry, or continue to eat after you are already satisfied, ask yourself why you ate and record your feelings next to what you ate. This record is the starting point for change. Once you know yourself and understand why you are eating when you are not hungry, you must come up with strategies for change.

Try also to identify the types of food you often turn to when eating emotionally. An insatiable desire for sweets or fatty foods could signal an addiction or allergy. Watch for patterns. Some of us turn to food in times of stress. If this is the case, another strategy for dealing with stress must be learned. If loneliness or boredom is a catalyst for eating, you must focus on solving those problems.

A second strategy, which may be more effective, is to have an activity planned that will keep you busy and prevent you from thinking about food or eating. Rebekah realized that often she engaged in emotional eating when she was bored. She would come home from work and eat for entertainment. She decided to join a singles group at church and also to plan something to do every evening, be it installing a new printer, arranging a file drawer, or finishing a knitting project. She also planned enjoyable events with friends or the church group, such as yoga class, swimming, or just getting together to socialize. These activities not only kept her away from food, but helped her increase physical activity, further assisting weight loss. Once Rebekah lost the first five or ten pounds, the rewards began to encourage her even more, and the habit of eating each evening was broken.

As a trigger for eating, stress is a little more difficult to predict and to establish a plan for combating. Stress really does increase chemicals in the brain that cause us to desire food—especially unhealthy food. According to a study published in the April 2004 *Endocrinology,* we produce cortisol when we are under stress, and cortisol stimulates the production of neuropeptide Y, which activates carbohydrate cravings. This same neuropeptide also causes the body to retain and store the new body fat that we produce. In addition, increased cortisol increases insulin, and high insulin leads to fat storage and retention. Thus, chronic stress can increase your weight.

When stressful circumstances occur, you must be ready with strategies. You may have to try various strategies until you find one that works. It may be helpful to close your eyes and to breathe slowly and deeply to oxygenate and calm your body. Other strategies: sip a warm cup of chamomile tea, take a soothing bath by candlelight, play calming music, or exercise vigorously.

Another strategy is to substitute healthy food choices for the foods with which you habitually seek comfort. If you eat anything during an emotional situation, allow yourself only a piece of your favorite fruit or raw vegetables with dip. By substituting a healthier food, you can drastically reduce the negative, calorie-loading behavior. The ultimate goal is to discontinue the pattern of emotional eating, but this may be an effective first step. You also can make an affirmation along these lines: "I only eat when I am hungry." Repeat this whenever emotional eating tempts you. The counterpoint to emotional eating is to *identify* the specific emotions that trigger your eating and *plan* tactics for conquering those triggers. Understanding all this about yourself is key to your freedom from food domination.

Don't Discount the Power of Prayer

We are not just bodies and minds; we are beings with a spiritual nature. Spirituality takes different forms for different people, but when that side of a person is ignored—when we neglect meditation and prayer—we miss a vital aspect of life and health. Scientific evidence confirms the correlation between physical health and "religion," spirituality, and prayer. Most people in today's society, however, do not consider spirituality as a necessary component for optimal health. They would probably be surprised to hear that their spiritual side is a key ally in weight loss, but we have seen the evidence time and again; the peace, joy, fulfillment, and contentment that accompany meditation and prayer are powerful healing agents. While science can not fully fathom the mystery of why or how prayer is so powerful in health and healing, studies and thousands of years of human history indicate that it is. In its simplest form, prayer can be defined as *intention* and *attention.* Similar to affirmations, the essence of prayer is giving attention to something along with a strong intention.

Larry Dossey, in his book *Healing Words,* reports one remarkable 1988 study undertaken by Dr. Randolph Byrd, a cardiologist at San Francisco General Hospital. In this study, 393 coronary care patients at the hospital were divided into two groups. One group, unbeknownst to them, was prayed for by home prayer groups while the other patients were not remembered in prayer. This was a double-blind study in which neither the patients nor their doctors and nurses knew the group assignments. The results were astounding. The group receiving prayer was five times less likely to require antibiotics, three times less likely to develop pulmonary edema, and not one required a ventilator, while twelve in the other group did. Additionally, fewer deaths occurred in the group receiving the anonymous prayers. As if these facts were not amazing enough, we can only imagine how much more effective the prayer may have been if the patients were aware of it or, even better, involved in the prayer groups. The encouragement provided by hearing the prayers of others on their behalf and pouring out their own minds and souls would seemingly have an even more powerful effect. Dossey calls prayer "one of the best-kept secrets in medical science."

Another positive outcome of prayer is that it often takes our minds off of ourselves and our problems and causes us to focus on the needs of others. When we stop being so self-involved by realizing and praying for the needs of others, it often leads to actively reaching out to help others. At times this transfer of mental and physical energy alone brings positive physical rewards.

If you have a friend or group of friends who are also trying to change their lifestyle, why not join together and pray with and for each other? When you are tempted to eat unhealthy foods, pray for strength to resist. During workouts, meditation and prayer can pass the time and lift your thoughts from the hard work.

Laugh Off a Few of Those Extra Pounds

An equally powerful provider of health and wellness—including weight loss—is laughter. Ancient wisdom says that a cheerful heart is like good medicine. Science is proving this to be valid. Norman Cousins's book *Anatomy of an Illness* describes how he brought about his own amazing recovery from ankylosing spondylitis (a connective tissue disease) using laughter as a key component. Cousins discovered that ten minutes of genuine, hearty laughter would ease his pain for hours. He used funny movies to ignite laughter, sparking profound health benefits.

The inspiring movie *Patch Adams,* based on the true story of a medical student, illustrates how humor, happiness, and laughter are used with medicine to help children and adults recover. Britain's National Health Service actually opened a Laughter Clinic in the fall of 1991, and thousands of doctors, nurses, and medical professionals have trained there. There have been TV news stories on hospitals incorporating laughing rooms where patients can go to watch funny movies, read joke books, and enjoy laughter-provoking entertainment. Reports are that the patients who take advantage of these laughter rooms seem to have better chances of recovery and have quicker recoveries.

Most of us take life too seriously. The average child laughs about 150 times a day, while most adults laugh 10 or 15 times in a day. Robert Holden, a stress consultant, wrote an article published on the Internet called "A Dose of Laughter Medicine," in which he states, "We don't stop laughing because we grow old, we grow old because we stop laughing."

An exuberant belly laugh thoroughly exercises the hundreds of muscles, nerves, and organs in your core body. This exercise not only burns calories, but releases chemicals, including endorphins, throughout your system. These endorphins have a morphinelike effect, hence Norman Cousins's pain relief. They incite feelings of joy and well-being, giving us a natural high. Laughter lightens your mood, lifting stresses, discouragements, and tension. Further, your lungs absorb oxygen as you engage in hearty laughter, and your circulation is enhanced as blood vessels are opened. It is estimated that a prolonged period of laughter can increase blood flow equal to fifteen to thirty minutes of aerobic exercise. The science of psychoneuroimmunology, which is the fascinating study of how our state of mind affects our health, has shown that laughter even has a profound effect on the immune system. Just as suppressed anger, hatred, and bitterness hinder immune function, laughter supports the immune system. Research experiments of Drs. Lee Berk and Stanley Tan at Loma Linda University School of Medicine in California have shown that laughter stimulates the immune system to produce white cells called T cells, which prevent infection. Laughter was also proven to increase natural killer cells, which are lymphocytes that erode tumors and battle viruses, along with gamma interferon, a disease-fighting protein.

Laughing as part of a group can promote a sense of belonging and bonding. Brain function is improved as we indulge in regular laughter because it stimulates both sides of the brain, keeping us alert. Laughter helps us feel hopeful. Laughter energizes us, a clear benefit for those trying to lose weight. What better way to "exercise"?

The *NBFA* Lifestyle urges you to practice purposeful smiling and to find more ways to laugh. Become a "smile millionaire." Spend less time focusing on food and more time having fun. Since laughter is good for the cells, and healthy cells promote a healthy weight, learn to laugh again, find friends who make you laugh, and discover more joy in your life. In the process, you will most likely lose some pounds.

It's Your Move

Simply considering all the information in this chapter does nothing for your health or your weight. Only when you make a determined commitment to change your life do you improve.

For many people, losing weight is something they "should" do to be more acceptable to others. That is not the right motivation. Losing weight is about ensuring a longer life with your loved ones, living with less disability, and enjoying a higher quality of living. The choice is yours, and all the power you need—an amazing capacity—is within your own mind. You can settle for knowing without changing, or you can use the knowledge you have gained to create change in your life. You can liberate yourself from food addictions, emotional eating, and negative thoughts, and envision a slim, healthy, spiritually fulfilled, and positive new person who is energized by a spirit of happiness and laughter.

READER/CUSTOMER CARE SURVEY

HEFG

We care about your opinions! Please take a moment to fill out our online Reader Survey at **http://survey.hcibooks.com**.
As a **"THANK YOU"** you will receive a **VALUABLE INSTANT COUPON** towards future book purchases as well as a **SPECIAL GIFT** available only online! Or, you may mail this card back to us and we will send you a copy of our exciting catalog with your valuable coupon inside.

(PLEASE PRINT IN ALL CAPS)

First Name	MI.	Last Name

Address		

State	Zip	Email	City

1. Gender
❑ Female   ❑ Male

2. Age
❑ 8 or younger
❑ 9-12   ❑ 13-16
❑ 17-20   ❑ 21-30
❑ 31+

3. Did you receive this book as a gift?
❑ Yes   ❑ No

4. Annual Household Income
❑ under $25,000
❑ $25,000 - $34,999
❑ $35,000 - $49,999
❑ $50,000 - $74,999
❑ over $75,000

5. What are the ages of the children living in your house?
❑ 0 - 14   ❑ 15+

6. Marital Status
❑ Single
❑ Married
❑ Divorced
❑ Widowed

7. How did you find out about the book?
(please choose one)
❑ Recommendation
❑ Store Display
❑ Online
❑ Catalog/Mailing
❑ Interview/Review

8. Where do you usually buy books?
(please choose one)
❑ Bookstore
❑ Online
❑ Book Club/Mail Order
❑ Price Club (Sam's Club, Costco's, etc.)
❑ Retail Store (Target, Wal-Mart, etc.)

9. What subject do you enjoy reading about the most?
(please choose one)
❑ Parenting/Family
❑ Relationships
❑ Recovery/Addictions
❑ Health/Nutrition
❑ Christianity
❑ Spirituality/Inspiration
❑ Business Self-help
❑ Women's Issues
❑ Sports

10. What attracts you most to a book?
(please choose one)
❑ Title
❑ Cover Design
❑ Author
❑ Content

TAPE IN MIDDLE; DO NOT STAPLE

BUSINESS REPLY MAIL
FIRST-CLASS MAIL PERMIT NO 45 DEERFIELD BEACH, FL

POSTAGE WILL BE PAID BY ADDRESSEE

Health Communications, Inc.
3201 SW 15th Street
Deerfield Beach FL 33442-9875

FOLD HERE

Comments

THE PHYSICAL 8 PATHWAY

New Life—New Habits

O nce you have a healthy mind-set, you must move on to the powerful weapon of habits for maintaining the physical body. In this chapter you learn how physical activity— even spending time in the sun, sleeping, releasing stress, and breathing the right way—can help you to stay healthy and to lose weight. In this chapter, you'll discover:

- The benefits of physical activity, the many ways to work it into your life, and how to plan a strategy to implement it.

- The importance of other healthy habits such as exposure to sunshine, proper rest, stress release, and breathing exercises for health and weight loss.

- What a valuable tool the *NBFA* Journal can be, and how it will help keep you on track and provide accountability.
- How reading can motivate you and keep you on the right track.
- How regular fasting days can benefit your health and weight.

Teachers open the door, but you must enter by yourself.

—Chinese Proverb

Most of us have heard—often enough—that exercise is key to losing weight and keeping it off. And most of us have plenty of excuses why we can't find the time and energy to exercise. Once you understand the full scope of how what you *do* determines your health and your weight, we hope you will find it difficult to sit still.

This chapter gives you practical advice for tailoring your own plan for getting physical and moving toward health and weight loss. We've done the thinking. You just need to make it part of your life. Along the way you will also hear some surprising things about getting enough sun (we recommend you do that every day), getting enough sleep, reducing your stress, and learning how to breathe the right way. You will realize how all of that is important to staying trim. You will also learn why it is helpful, now and then, to stop eating completely; a fast can bring benefits you may never have envisioned.

Instant Gratification, Long-Term Consequence

Maintain a positive mind-set about changing your habits. Don't consider this negative, difficult, or drudgery. You are developing habits that will ultimately make you happy. As

Robert M. Pirsig, author of *Zen and the Art of Motorcycle Maintenance,* said, "It's so hard when contemplated in advance, and so easy when you do it." In *The Power of Focus,* authors Canfield, Hansen, and Hewitt state that, "If you keep on doing what you've always done, you'll keep on getting what you've always got." We encourage you to begin by tackling just one or two new healthy habits. If you incorporate healthy habits one day at a time, they soon become second-nature. Instead of sitting around thinking about how hard it is going to be, get off the couch, and get started. We are immersed in a culture programmed for immediate gratification—whether indulging in unhealthy food or watching television rather than exercising. Since outcomes are not felt instantaneously, the negative consequences down the road are often not considered up front. The habits that we build our lives upon today will greatly affect our health, happiness, and weight a month, a year, even five years from now.

In the remainder of this chapter, we will consider seven aspects of healthy living—exercise, sunshine, sleep, stress reduction, proper breathing, fasting, and journaling—in which you have the opportunity to build new routines, one at a time, that will bring you closer to health and further from overweight and diagnosable disease.

Your Body Burns Fat Even After Your Workout

There is an endless supply of excuses for why a person does not exercise: I don't have enough time. . . . I can't stand to sweat. . . . I am not athletic. . . . I cannot afford to join a gym. . . . I cannot afford to buy good equipment. . . . It is raining or snowing, or too cold or too hot.

We know that one key to losing weight and maintaining weight loss is physical activity—moving some or all of your 640-plus muscles—on a daily basis. Exercise trains your body to burn fat, and no weight-loss plan works in the long run without exercise. Many former yo-yo dieters have discovered that the way to keep weight off is to add exercise. You cannot lose weight if you are taking in more calories than you burn. Exercise also increases your body's production of growth hormone (which reduces fat storage), and physical activity wards off depression and binge eating.

A groundbreaking study reported in a 2005 issue of *Archives of Internal Medicine* found that regular exercisers added up to four years to their lifespan compared to sedentary people. Fortunately, gentle to moderate exercise is sufficient, but it must be regular. In fact, strenuous exercise may even cause you to lose less weight because you may end up eating more if you are doing high-intensity workouts. Exercise resets the body's metabolism, encouraging your body to burn more fat. In fact, the amount of fat you are burning right now and the amount of many beneficial chemicals being produced in your body depend on when and how you last exercised.

An obese person's body treats fats differently than the body of one who is physically fit. Two people can eat the same fats, but the obese person stores more fat. Exercise can change how an overweight person's body processes fats, altering the body's response from one of storing fat to burning fat. Substantially decreasing calories is not a solution and can actually cause the body to decrease its thyroid function and slow its metabolic rate in order to conserve energy. That is counterproductive to successful weight loss. By starving, one has less energy, does less exercise, and burns less fat, which results in unwanted pounds staying right where they are. Exercise and healthy eating habits are the answer.

While a regularly exercised body burns more fat, overweight individuals have to exercise longer if they want to lose weight rather than maintain their weight. For the first thirty minutes of exercise, the body burns available glucose (sugar). After about thirty minutes, glucose is reduced and the body starts to burn fat instead of sugar. Overweight people need to build up to where they are able to exercise for longer than thirty minutes at a time in order to burn fat.

Another benefit of exercise is that energy expenditure remains elevated even after you finish your workout. Aerobic activity causes your metabolic rate to increase not only while engaging in activity, but for several hours afterward. Weight training is even more impressive. It increases your metabolic rate for up to two days after training. This means your body burns more calories and you lose more weight!

Yo-Yo Dieters: Listen Up

Coauthor Michelle was, for many years, a classic yo-yo dieter. She remembers being on a diet most of the time between the ages of thirteen and thirty-four.

I tried every sort of diet imaginable. I lost the same twenty-five pounds over and over again and gained it back every time. Never in my life had I *consistently* exercised. I got on exercise kicks now and then, but it never became a daily habit. I remember bragging that I was not the type to exercise because I hated to sweat. All of that changed when I was thirty-four. I lost the same twenty-five pounds again, but this time I began walking daily. After a while, my weight hit a plateau, so I began to run as far as I could, walking intermittently. I did this until I was running two miles at a time without stopping. That was what it took to resume weight loss, and I got down to my goal weight for the first time ever. This gave me a whole new attitude about exercise, and I began to run more, usually three or four miles a day. I finally got the correlation between how much I exercised and my weight, and I began to enjoy exercise.

At age forty, I ran a relay marathon, doing the 7.5-mile leg. My body learned to sweat effectively, and I realized that exercise made me feel better physically and mentally. I don't like it when I must miss a day for any reason. I don't *always* run. As I became physically fit and more educated, I expanded my workouts. Three days a week I do light weight lifting. Some days I enjoy rebounding, dancing, spinning, stair climbing, the elliptical trainer, swimming, bike riding, roller blading, or brisk walking. New habits helped me to expand my interests. I enjoy hiking more than watching television. I would rather take a bike ride than sit and watch a movie.

The more you get moving, the more agile your body becomes, opening the door for enjoying new activities. I am now forty-four, and I feel and look better than I did when I was in my twenties. I went from a size 12 to a size 4. College friends have told me I seem to be looking younger all the time. I am happy to say that I feel younger too—exercise, along with a nutrient-rich diet, made the difference for me. Along the way, I learned how to eat a cellularly healthy diet, based mainly on fresh, raw vegetables and fruits. I never gained those twenty-five pounds back! I will never have to lose them again! Success was finally achieved by incorporating physical activity along with a healthy diet. Exercise is *essential*.

Exercise: The Ultimate Anti-Aging Beauty Secret

Physical activity keeps you looking and feeling young. Those who stay active—riding bicycles, hiking, swimming, gardening, walking, and enjoying adventures of all kinds—appear younger than their years.

Exercise guru Jack La Lanne celebrated his ninetieth birthday in 2004. He is a great example of physical fitness leading to longevity. To celebrate his seventieth birthday, La Lanne swam, handcuffed and shackled, towing seventy boats with seventy people from the Queen's Way Bridge in Long Beach Harbor to the *Queen Mary,* a distance of one and a half miles. When his star was unveiled on the Hollywood Walk of Fame on his eighty-eighth birthday, he celebrated by doing eighty-eight pushups. Physical activity keeps you young, and a sedentary life makes you old before your time. That is a guarantee.

Understanding how vital exercise is to health, weight loss, and longevity serves as a motivator. Beginning to see positive changes in yourself will add to your motivation. When your motivation wanes, consider the long list of health benefits that come from physical activity, or better yet, copy the box on page 188 and post it where you can read it daily.

The Number of Benefits Is Astounding

Our cells need physical activity in order to stay healthy. Our lymphatic system gathers and removes waste from our 75 trillion cells, but it does not have a pump. While the heart serves as a pump for the circulatory system, the lymphatic system is dependent upon physical movement. Our bodies have three times as much lymph as blood. When we are inactive, toxins back up in our cells and cannot be eliminated, and that leads to disease. (One of the most effective exercises for moving lymph in our cells is rebounding, which is bouncing up and down on a mini-trampoline. We'll talk about that later in this chapter.)

Consider the dozens of other ways that exercise not only helps to keep off unwanted weight, but is essential to overall health, well-being, and appearance.

EXERCISE IMPROVES APPEARANCE:
• Helps maintain youthfulness/vitality
• Promotes weight loss/muscle mass
• Tightens sagging skin
• Increases balance/coordination

EXERCISE IMPROVES MENTAL/EMOTIONAL STATE:
• Promotes positive outlook/reduces depression
• Brings clarity of mind/better mental functioning
• Reduces stress

EXERCISE PROMOTES OVERALL HEALTH:
• Prevents both causes of disease—deficiency and toxicity
• Promotes delivery of nutrients to cells
• Pumps toxins out of the body
• Boosts the immune system and oxygenates cells

EXERCISE PROMOTES WEIGHT LOSS:
• Key to permanent weight loss
• Burns fat
• Increases muscle, which also burns more fat
• Speeds metabolism/reduces sluggishness
• Decreases appetite
• Promotes efficient, regular elimination
• Promotes better sleep

EXERCISE PREVENTS MANIFESTATIONS OF DISEASE:
• Improves digestion
• Lowers blood pressure
• Dissolves blood clots
• Strengthens the heart
• Improves circulation
• Strengthens bones and joints
• Reduces cancer risk
• Stabilizes blood sugar
• Promotes quicker healing

Vary Your Exercise Routine

To get the most benefit from your exercise program, include three different types of exercise: aerobic, weight-bearing, and stretching/flexibility movements.

Aerobic—also referred to as cardiovascular—exercise gets the body warmed up, the heart pumping, the blood circulating, and the oxygen flowing more rapidly into and out of the lungs. Aerobic exercises include jogging, rebounding, elliptical training, stair climbing, bicycling, speed walking, fitness classes, dance, and so on. This type of exercise burns fat and calories, helps circulate the lymph, and increases oxygen supply to the tissues. It is essential to weight loss, but also critical for health, helping to prevent cancer and heart disease.

Walking is something almost anyone can do, and it is an effective low-impact aerobic exercise. Walking doesn't require training, is easy on the joints, and is of significant value. If you are in poor shape, start out with slow-paced walking. Regardless of where you begin, the faster you walk and the longer the distance, the greater the benefits. A two-year study of two hundred overweight people was reported in the October 24, 2005, edition of *USA Today.* The study found that those who walked briskly an average of at least forty minutes a day lost the most weight. It also showed that those who listened to their favorite music while walking followed the exercise plan more closely and lost about twice as much weight as those who didn't.

Weight or resistance training increases muscular strength and endurance. It also helps promote healthy bones, joints, and tissues—preventing arthritis and osteoporosis. Diet alone will never resolve or prevent osteoporosis; weight-bearing exercise is essential to build bone density. Seek guidance as you undertake resistance exercise because proper technique is imperative. Smooth, controlled movements and correct form are essential for maximum benefit and injury prevention.

Before, during, and after exercise, stretching can prevent tight, rigid tissues, which are more susceptible to injury. Stretching makes your workout easier and more comfortable and helps prevent muscle soreness. Flexibility is increased with ongoing stretching. Do not overlook this healthy part of your workout.

Rebounding: So Easy and So Effective

Rebounding is a fun and unique exercise that involves bouncing up and down on a mini-trampoline—and its effects are almost magical. It is enjoyable and so easy to do. It can be done by almost anyone regardless of age or physical condition. Rebounding sounds too good to be true, but it tones, conditions, strengthens, and heals the entire body in as little as fifteen minutes a day. Six minutes of rebounding is estimated to be equivalent to one mile of jogging.

Why are we so excited about rebounding? Because it is remarkably therapeutic for cells. Research presented in 2000 at the annual meeting of the American Thoracic Society found that physically moving cells has a profound impact on their biochemistry and behavior. Moving and stretching cells—as rebounding does—helps to supply essential nutrients and to eliminate toxic waste products. When you bounce on a rebounder, your entire body (internal organs, bones, connective tissue, and skin) becomes stronger, more flexible, and healthier. Blood circulation and lymphatic drainage are vastly improved.

To picture the effect that rebounding has on cells, visualize a balloon filled with water. Hold the balloon by its stem and observe how gravity pulls on the water, slightly stretching the balloon. While you are still holding the balloon, move your hand rapidly up and down and observe how the extra gravitational force causes the balloon to significantly stretch and distort. When you bounce up and down on a rebounder, this is what happens to every cell in your body. When cells are exercised in this way brain function is improved, muscle is built, metabolism is increased, fat is burned, tissues are healed, blood pressure is regulated, appetite is curbed, balance and coordination are enhanced, and fatigue is eliminated. Rebounding builds stronger bones and joints, improves immunity and healing, tightens skin, resolves back problems, improves vision and hearing, and stabilizes the nervous system, reducing stress. Rebounding also improves digestion and elimination and increases oxygen uptake, promoting detoxification through the lungs, skin, and lymph systems.

Weight training is great exercise, but it applies weight and movement only to a particular muscle or set of muscles at one time. You do one exercise to work the triceps, another for the quadriceps, and a different routine for the pectorals. Rebounding is a more efficient way of exercising your entire body because it applies weight and movement to every cell. The extra force of gravity caused by bouncing on the mat strengthens bones and joints without jarring impact.

Dr. James White from the University of California, San Diego, and author of *Jump for Joy* says that rebounding is "the closest thing to the Fountain of Youth that science has discovered," and that it "is effective in improving the symptoms of over 80% of the patients reporting to our rehabilitation lab." Even patients in their nineties have experienced remarkable improvement. Rebounders are sold with a stabilizing bar for those concerned about balance. Bouncing chairs are available for wheelchair-bound or incapacitated individuals so that the upper half of the body is still able to derive great benefit from this exercise.

Aside from the health benefits, rebounding is convenient since you can do it at home, indoors, or outdoors. You can purchase a rebounder that is foldable and comes with a carrying case so it is easily transported. You can do several short rebounding sessions or one longer one. Any amount of time spent rebounding provides benefits. If you are unable to do long sessions, bouncing for two minutes every hour can be beneficial. For an aerobic workout, the time and intensity must be adjusted to accommodate your fitness level. You can take advantage of the time spent rebounding to listen to educational audio or video tapes, watch television, move to your favorite music, or even work out with one of the many rebounding videos available.

When purchasing a rebounder, do not buy a cheap forty-dollar mini-trampoline at a sporting goods store. It may look the same as a high-quality rebounder at first glance, but this type of rebounder can do more harm than good. The cheap tube springs found on most mini-trampolines do not absorb and cushion your weight properly. You can suffer permanent nerve damage on rebounders that are not well built. Double, fat-barrel springs allow for smooth deceleration, and a high-quality mat is necessary for proper support (see Appendix D for recommendations).

Tips to Keep You on Track

As you incorporate exercise into every day, remember these tips to help you sustain your healthy new habits:

1. **Start at your own pace.** If you have never exercised, begin with a ten- or fifteen-minute walk every day and build gradually. Do not overdo at the outset. Overexercising at the beginning will cause soreness and discouragement.

2. **Schedule time for exercise each day.** Make an appointment in your plan book that you do not break. If it is not scheduled, it may not happen. Having a consistent daily time will help you to make it part of your routine. Strive to build up to more than thirty minutes of exercise a day as you are able. Exercise can be accomplished at any time during the day, but morning is

preferable for many because if a workout is put off until later in the day it may be squeezed out by a demanding schedule or cancelled due to weariness. You have more energy in the morning. If you exercise before you have eaten, you burn fat as you exercise, rather than the food you have recently eaten.

3. **Choose an exercise that you enjoy.** You are far more likely to continue exercising if you find pleasure in the activity. The variety is expansive, so try different forms of exercise until you find one or a few that you can maintain.

4. **Exercise does not require expensive equipment or gym memberships.** It can be as simple as getting out for a daily walk. Quality walking shoes are the only requirement. Work at walking until you can walk a mile in fifteen minutes. This pace is challenging. Once you can do that, try two miles in thirty minutes, building up to four miles in an hour.

5. **Find an exercise partner.** The accountability and companionship provided by a buddy make your exercise time more consistent and pleasurable. On days when you don't feel like working out, your partner can spur you on. If money is not a problem, hire a trainer to motivate and direct you.

6. **Post and review the benefits of exercise daily.** Seek to maintain a positive attitude toward your daily exercise. Remind yourself of the ways this new habit is making you healthier. While you exercise, visualize the healthier, thinner you that will result.

7. **Vary your exercise routines so you don't get bored.** Walk in different locations so that you can enjoy the scenery of new places. Have indoor routines planned for rainy days. Turn on the music and dance, go to an exercise class, or jump on your rebounder.

8. **Do not relegate exercise only to your planned time.**
   Incorporate more movement into your entire day. Any
   and all activity is helpful. Think of practical ways to
   increase activity. Run your own errands instead of sending your child; use the steps rather than an elevator or
   escalator; don't drive around looking for a closer park-
   ing spot; take a break from sedentary work and do some
   jumping jacks, rebound for a couple minutes, or do
   pushups to get your blood moving. Put some extra
   bounce into daily, routine activities—turn on music and
   dance as you do household chores.

9. **Do not allow yourself to sit in front of the television
   night after night.** If you want to watch a program,
   rebound while you watch or pedal on a stationary
   bicycle. Or do exercises during commercial breaks—
   pushups during one break, situps during the next, then
   perhaps stretching for the third.

10. *Reward yourself in some way for every week of consis-
    tent daily exercise.* Providing such encouragement is
    especially important at the outset. Allow yourself to
    indulge in a special activity (besides eating). You can
    even plan some sort of reward with your exercise part-
    ner to motivate both of you.

Add your own tips to this list. The important thing is to get
yourself moving and to do it today. Sixty percent of the adult
population in our country is sedentary. Don't allow yourself to
be part of that deadly statistic.

Don't Block Out the Sun

The media and others in our society, including most of our
physicians, tell us that the sun's rays are harmful. They
instruct us to lather up with sunscreen and put it on our babies
and children. People have been so frightened by all of the

press about skin cancer that many avoid the sun as their worst enemy. But think about it. Did our ancestors use sunscreen? Did they stay out of the sun? Most of them were outdoors every day, and they did not suffer the cancer and other chronic diseases that we do. The truth is that our bodies need sunlight, which is an essential and highly beneficial nutrient. Too much food is harmful to your body, and too much sun can be harmful as well. But full-spectrum sunlight, in the proper amount, is vital to your health. Sunlight feels good on your skin and makes you feel good. It helps your mood in general, and it also helps to control food cravings. Sunlight helps to lower blood sugar and insulin, which helps to control weight. It also reduces the resting heart rate (lessening the workload on the heart). Sunlight increases the body's ability to deal with stress, lowers blood pressure, boosts the immune system, and helps keep hormones balanced. The sun draws toxins out of your body through the skin. Sunlight helps your body produce vitamin D. It is one of the few sources of vitamin D, which is essential for strong and healthy bones and for preventing cancer, multiple sclerosis, and other diseases.

A study published in the January–February 2005 issue of *Psychosomatic Medicine* assigned some patients who were recovering from spinal surgery to sunny rooms while others were given rooms on the darker side of the hospital. The patients who were recovering in the sunny rooms reported less stress and used 22 percent less painkiller per hour than the patients in the darker rooms. Serotonin is increased in the brain with sunlight exposure, and this chemical has an impact on mood, appetite, and sleep. This, at least partly, explains the study's outcome.

Make wise choices as you begin to make sunlight a regular routine. The sun's rays are the hottest between the hours of 11:00 AM and 3:00 PM. We have been advised to avoid the sun during those hours, which is poor advice, because the specific wavelengths required to produce vitamin D are at their peak during those hours. Vitamin D is now one of our population's biggest deficiencies because people are avoiding the sun. While we must avoid sun*burn*, which results from excessive or inconsistent exposure to the sun, sun *exposure* during these peak hours is especially beneficial for acquiring vitamin D. Begin by allowing your skin (especially if you are fair) to be exposed to sunlight for ten to fifteen minutes a day. Slowly and cautiously increase time in the sun, occasionally soaking in thirty minutes at a time on as much of your body as possible. The darker your natural skin, the more important it is that you obtain sunshine during peak hours and for a longer time. Fair-skinned individuals, whose ancestors originated in northern climates with less sun, will get all the vitamin D they need in a much shorter time and must to be careful not to burn.

If you have to be in the sun for longer periods, do not use commercial sunscreens that are toxic, which is virtually all of them. Some of the chemicals in these lotions are toxic in and of themselves while others undergo chemical change when exposed to the sun after application, forming cancer-causing compounds on your skin. Sunscreen may thus contribute to skin cancer rather than helping you to avoid it. It may not be a coincidence that skin cancer rates have increased as the use of sunscreens and other body creams and lotions has increased. In fact, skin cancer rates are the highest among populations that use the most sunscreen. Meanwhile skin cancer is rare in many third-world countries where sunscreen is not used and long hours are spent working outdoors.

Better alternatives for protection during longer periods in the sun are available, nutrition being the best. Fresh vegetables and fruits, which are the building blocks of the *NBFA* Lifestyle, provide a goldmine of antioxidant protection for your skin, making it more resistant to sun damage. Once you are living the *NBFA* Lifestyle and increasing your raw vegetable and fruit consumption, you will eventually notice an increase in the amount of time you can be in the sun safely.

Carotenes, which are found in colorful vegetables and fruits such as carrots, sweet potatoes, bell peppers, squash, cantalope, papaya, and others, protect the skin from sunlight, and are often called "nature's sun umbrella." In *The Sunfood Diet Success System,* raw-fooder David Wolfe states, "The benefits of sunshine are improved by eating correctly. . . . When the body is clean and internally protected with beta-carotene you will be amazed at how long you can be in the sun and how well you tan. When people eat correctly and are detoxified, exposure to the sun cannot lead to skin cancer."

Another option for sun protection is to rub high-quality olive oil or coconut oil on your skin. The oil must be of such quality that it still contains adequate antioxidants (see Appendix D for recommendations). Using olive oil to protect the skin was an ancient custom in the Mediterranean and is practiced by many Mediterranean people today. Modern research shows that olive oil will even help to repair skin after it has been burned.

Another sensible alternative is to dissolve vitamin C powder in a small amount of water or in a safe skin cream and apply the mixture to your skin. About a 10 percent solution works well. If you are just beginning to use the vitamin C, it is best to reapply it after being in the water to optimize the amount of vitamin C in your cells. As you continue to use it, protective levels will build up in your skin and you won't need to reapply it after swimming. Vitamin C is absorbed into the cells and is still present up to thirty-six hours after it has been applied topically to the skin. In addition to protecting your skin from burning, vitamin C is good for your skin in general, helping to keep it in good repair.

It's Not a Tabloid Headline: Lose Weight While You Sleep

Millions of Americans are walking around sleep deprived, contributing to our epidemic of overweight.

According to the National Institutes of Health, growing evidence links chronic lack of sleep to increased risk of obesity, as well as diabetes, heart disease, and infections. Recent news stories have highlighted the fact that you can lose weight just by sleeping more. Sleep deprivation decreases the level of the hormone leptin, a hormone that helps you feel satiated. Sleep-deprived people, therefore, feel more compelled to eat. Sleep deprivation also increases levels of the hormone ghrelin, a hormone that encourages appetite. Sleep-deprived individuals also often try to compensate for their fatigue by eating more. When the body lacks energy, it is a natural, though often unconscious, response to seek energy by eating. Unfortunately, the types of foods that are usually craved—coffee, sugar, chocolate, and other stimulants—damage cells and add excess calories.

When sleep deprivation is a pattern, our chemical and hormonal balance is thrown out of whack, resulting in weight gain and a compromised immune system. A shortage of sleep unbalances the hormones cortisol, human growth hormone (HGH), and prolactin. Elevated cortisol damages brain cells, resulting in forgetfulness and a spaced-out feeling. Cortisol also causes the body to gain weight by increasing both appetite and fat storage. Both HGH and prolactin are beneficial hormones that are produced during sleep. HGH is needed to repair and rebuild damaged tissue. Prolactin enhances immune response, and a deficiency leaves us vulnerable to infection. Studies have shown that losing even one night of sleep can impair immunity, and a week of interrupted sleep patterns is enough to create hormonal chaos, inviting disease.

Not too many generations ago, people could not work after

dark. Life mostly shut down when the sun went down, providing more time for sleep. Today, most of us live in cities that never sleep. Sleep experts recommend seven to nine hours of sleep per night for adults, but 40 percent of our adult population gets less. Multitudes have forgotten what it feels like to be truly rested. To keep up with the demands of life, sleep is sacrificed even though being deprived of sleep actually causes us to be much less productive. Data released in March 2006 by the National Sleep Foundation concluded that only one in five children is getting the recommended nine hours of sleep, which is causing 28 percent of our high school students to fall asleep in class. Students getting more sleep achieve higher grades.

Think about your personal energy level. Are you lethargic and fatigued most of the time? Do you drag yourself out of bed and find it a chore to make it through the day, often listless and dependent upon artificial stimulants such as coffee and sugar? Energy levels are actually an excellent barometer of health. Boundless natural energy is a general indicator that your cells are functioning well. Continual fatigue is your body's cry for help. During the hours you sleep, your body has time and energy to remove toxins, a vital process for health and well-being. Sleep is also the prime time for your body to recharge itself, build new cells, repair damaged ones, and replenish cellular energy. If we are giving our bodies the raw materials they require for building healthy cells, we certainly want to give them the down time that they need to get the job done.

Stress May Make You Store More Fat

Although some people may think that stress can cause weight loss, in reality reducing stress is important to your health and to permanent weight control. The immediate response to acute stress can be a loss of appetite and weight loss, but chronic stress increases appetite and fat storage, making you fat.

Our bodies naturally produce certain hormones in stressful circumstances. These hormones, such as adrenalin and cortisol, are what we call fight-or-flight hormones and are designed to provide a rush of strength to deal with an emergency. The way they prepare the body for action is by increasing blood pressure and heart rate. Our bodies were designed to deal with these hormones in rare crisis situations. When stress is chronic, as it is for many people, these reactions damage cells and impair health, contributing to overweight.

An overabundance of stress chemicals can cause problems: immune problems, poor digestion (which affects weight loss), sleep disturbance (which affects weight loss), water retention (which adds weight), fat deposits (which add weight), hypo-glycemia (a disease related to how we metabolize sugar), decreased bone and muscle mass, ulcers, anxiety, fatigue, depression, high blood pressure, cardiovascular problems, and on top of all of that, an increase in appetite. Stressful situations alone are not harmful; the harm results from inappropriate reactions to stressors. Whether the challenge is mental, physical, or emotional, you need to find coping strategies to reduce your anxiety and stress. In today's world, stress, more often than not, is chronic rather than occasional. People are working more, sleeping less, and leading lives that are too fast-paced and overwhelming.

You have the ability to reduce some of those sources of stress and also to control your responses to stress. Much of the battle lies in believing you are able to deal with each situation. We can choose not to become upset about things that we have no power to change, such as a traffic backup or the rude actions of other drivers. Though the physical responses to stress, such as increased heart rate, are automatic, they do not act independently of the mind. Changing your focus to positive thoughts can have a significant effect. Relax, try some deep breathing, and regain your composure. Once you understand how damaging stress chemicals are to your health, you may find more strength to choose composure.

Stress can also trigger unhealthy behaviors, from nail-biting to smoking, drinking, or overeating. Your first step is to recognize what behavior you resort to in dealing with stress. Most overweight individuals rush to comfort foods, whether sweets (looking for a sugar high) or crunchy, salty indulgences. Such foods are not only poor nutrition choices, but the body is not able to properly digest them during stressful circumstances. Physical exercise is a healthy alternative, using up the hormones produced during stress. If you absolutely must eat, choose a nutritious snack such as raw vegetables with a healthy dip or a piece of fruit. You won't be facing the letdown and guilt that follow a sugar high or a fatty indulgence.

A nutritious diet and proper supplements, particularly the B vitamins, can lessen the negative effects of stress. Green leafy vegetables, such as romaine, spinach, kale, Swiss chard, and leaf lettuce, are good choices. Make time for healthy meals, no matter how tight your schedule. Do not overcommit yourself to the point that meals are rushed or skipped.

Just Breathe—But Be Careful Where and How

Did you know that 96 percent of the nutrients your body uses every day are acquired from the air that you breathe rather than from the food you eat? Think about it: you can go days without food and even water, but you cannot go for more than a few minutes without oxygen. Oxygen is the cell's most vital nutrient. Inhaling high-quality air in order to maintain our health is something we rarely consider, yet it can drastically affect how we look and feel, our resistance to disease, and even how long we live.

Deep breathing of fresh air is an essential part of health maintenance and weight loss. Oxygenating your cells energizes your body. The more oxygen available to your cells, the more energetic and less hungry you will feel. The next time you are hungry or tired, take a few minutes outside to practice deep breathing. Your appetite will likely be suppressed and your sluggishness diminished.

Be sure to check two things, though: the quality of air that you breathe and the manner in which you breathe. The healthiest air is found in wooded areas or at the seashore, but almost all outdoor air is better than indoor air. The EPA calls indoor air pollution the nation's worst environmental health problem, estimating that it is two to ten times as bad as outdoor air pollution. With the latest technology in thermal windows and doors, homes today are more airtight than ever. Most families unknowingly use many toxins in their household daily. Carpets, furnishings, gas-fired appliances, and household cleaning products all contribute. Airtight windows—along with central air conditioning and heating systems that recirculate air—keep toxins inside. This polluted air may cause headaches, eye irritations, breathing difficulties, respiratory congestion, cough, and asthma—all symptoms of unhealthy cells.

Another contributor to the low quality of indoor air is the loss of its negative charge. Fresh outdoor air, whether in the mountains or at the seashore, has a negative electrical charge, usually two thousand to four thousand negative ions per cubic centimeter. The negative ions in most indoor environments are between one hundred and two hundred per cubic centimeter. Air that is recirculated over and over again in homes and buildings loses its negative charge. In his book *Proof Positive,* Dr. Neil Nedley delineates many physical effects of breathing air with negative ions. He cites a change in brain chemistry leading to a more positive mood, lower blood pressure, and fewer ulcers as just a few. He says that "normal children and those with learning disabilities showed measurable improvements in brain function"—all of this from breathing negatively charged air.

The quality of the air that we breathe as we sleep also is

vital to our health. Ideally you should sleep with your windows open, even if only a crack, to allow fresh air into the room where you spend the most time. While this is easier to do in temperate areas, even northerners can keep their window opened slightly during most of the winter. Once you adjust to the fresh air, you won't want to sleep without it.

Another consideration is an air purifier, especially for individuals with chemical sensitivities, asthma, or allergy problems. Some critically ill clients have discovered that their illnesses were due, in large part, to the toxic air that they were breathing. Dr. Flora Van Orden, a representative for the Physician's Committee for Responsible Medicine, told us how ill she became just after moving to a new home in California. The home was located adjacent to an area where tractor-trailers stopped for the night, resulting in toxic diesel fumes. Unaware that this was the reason for her new health problems, which included headaches and coughing with excess mucus, her doctors initially believed the source was viral. Puzzled, the doctors then decided the cause was chronic obstructive pulmonary disease (COPD). The only relief they could offer her was in the form of prescription drugs and inhalers. Flora suffered these symptoms for a year. When her teaching contract expired, she moved from the area, and within three days her symptoms were gone. Flora's story is representative of thousands. Some readers may be having health issues that neither they nor their physicians have thought to trace, simply, to the air they are breathing.

In addition to the quality of the air you breathe there is actually a right way—a healthy way—and a wrong way to breathe. Most people are not aware that they are breathing the wrong way, although it is simple to change your ways. Effective breathing is accomplished by using the diaphragm, a deep abdominal muscle intended for breathing. When you are using your diaphragm, you are doing "belly breathing" rather than chest breathing. It is an effortless and efficient way to breathe.

Take note of how you are breathing right now. Are you using your upper back and chest as you inhale? Many people breathe this way, and it is much more difficult. When you breathe with the diaphragm, you are breathing downward and your stomach (guts) move out and away, making more room for the lungs to fill deeply with air. This technique enhances the function of your entire respiratory system. Each breath should begin downward in the belly.

Correct breathing should also be through the nose (which acts as a filter), rather than the mouth, and breathing should be rather slow. While you are resting, you should take less than fifteen breaths per minute. Eight to ten breaths per minute is ideal.

Here is a simple test to see how you are doing: Lie on your back on the floor, put a book on your abdomen, breathe through your nose, and watch to see if the book goes up and down with each breath. Concentrate on proper belly breathing until the book moves up and down. Once you begin breathing this way, be sure to incorporate it while exercising. Next, count the number of breaths you take in a minute. Try to limit the count to less than fifteen and, preferably, less than ten.

A good habit to integrate into your daily schedule is to do deep breathing exercises. Take a few minutes in the morning and again in the evening to seek out fresh air and take ten to twenty breaths using techniques such as this one.

Inhale for five counts, hold the air for five counts, exhale for five counts, and then wait with no air for five counts. You can choose any number of seconds. Choose what works best and is most comfortable for you.

Begin to practice with five breaths, and build up to ten or twenty. Close your breathing exercise routine by taking a few deep breaths in, stretching the arms upward and out, slowly bringing them back down again.

If you are feeling stressed, tired, or hungry, take a short break, go outdoors and do a few breathing exercises. This is one excellent weight-loss habit!

Give Your Body a Break—From Food

Another strategy that is part of the *NBFA* Lifestyle is to take a rest completely from eating—to fast. The human body was designed to deal with periods of not eating at all. Our hunter-gatherer ancestors fasted because food was not always available. Fasting, or giving the body a rest from food, is one of the oldest and most effective healing methods. We fast every night, which is why we call the first meal of the day "break fast." Time without food moving through the digestive system is critical to our health. Because our cells do not have to devote energy to the hard work of digestion, they can tap into energy needed for detoxification, maintenance, and healing. Giving your body additional periods of fasting besides overnight is a healthy habit to add to your lifestyle. Time without food means fewer calories, which supports weight loss, and this resting period allows for many healthful body functions that support weight loss and weight maintenance.

Whether you begin by fasting through just one meal a day, two meals a day, one day a week, or three days a month, your body will have extra time to cleanse and detoxify. Several studies suggest that fasting extends longevity. The late Dr. Roy Walford, coauthor of *The Retardation of Aging and Disease by Dietary Restriction,* did a study in which he fasted mice. His study showed that the mice that fasted two days a week *doubled* their life span and were healthier. Fasting is reported to cause healing, sometimes incredible healing for problems ranging from asthma to cancer, as well as other benefits such as lowered cholesterol and blood pressure, reduction in sleeping problems, a slowing of the aging process, and improved elimination. Additionally, fasting can help improve or eliminate food and drug addictions, including nicotine addiction. Patricia Bragg, a health educator, consultant, and crusader, calls fasting "nature's cure."

In his book *Juice Fasting and Detoxification,* Steve

Meyerowitz states, "One- and three-day fasts are wonderful for breaking the cycle of binges, cravings, sweets and other bad patterns or habits. . . . When it comes to losing weight, sensible fasting has no equal. Results are dramatic and can be lasting if you use it as an opportunity to break from poor eating habits. By consuming higher-quality foods, the body will get the nutrients it needs and not think it is starving even when it is getting fewer calories. Not only that, short-term fasting is completely natural and superior to pills and drugs with all their undesirable side effects. The only side effects you get with fasting are a drop in high blood pressure along with the pounds."

Fasting one day a week is not difficult, and will give your body fifty-two days a year to rest, detoxify, and repair. The main reason for this habit is health, but it also helps to lose weight as fewer calories are consumed. As fasting helps your body eliminate toxins, you will notice increased energy, better health, and sharper mental functioning.

There are different kinds of fasts. A simple water fast is one in which all you consume is water. Pure water helps to flush toxins through your system as your body releases them. A water fast that includes buffered vitamin C powder stirred into the water provides extra antioxidant power to protect from free radicals, and vitamin C also helps the body to detoxify. Some people, wishing to detoxify faster, drink excessive amounts of water. Excessive anything is not a good idea.

In another type of fast, you drink only fresh, home-juiced vegetables. In addition to these juices, you must drink plenty of pure water and lemon water. In the case of a juice fast, you may have a little more energy, which can be helpful if you are expending a lot of energy during the fast. The vegetable juice also provides nutrients to afford protection from the toxins that are released into your system as your body detoxifies.

Organic lemon juice in pure water during fasting can be helpful in the cleansing process, especially in supporting the liver. Your liver is the main organ in the detoxification process since toxins are collected in and flushed through the liver. Lemon acts as a stimulant to the liver, helping it to cleanse. The juice of one organic lemon mixed with sixteen to twenty-four ounces of pure water and consumed in the morning assists the liver. Since lemon is also a valuable source of vitamin C, this powerful antioxidant is available to neutralize free radicals that are released in the body during the fast. If you desire to make fasting a habit, an excellent book to reference is *Toxic Relief* by Dr. Don Colbert.

We encourage you, however, to start fasting only after you are well under way with other healthy lifestyle changes. Making too many changes at first will bring on a rapid detoxification, which may not only sicken you, but may also discourage you. There are also some individuals who should not fast because of blood-sugar problems. If you suffer with hypoglycemia or diabetes, these issues should be remedied before you pursue fasting. To keep blood sugar stable, such individuals need to eat regularly. Without food at regular intervals, insulin swings can provoke dizziness, fatigue, perspiration, lightheadedness, shakiness, headaches, and other symptoms. The good news is that type 2 diabetes and hypoglycemia are very easily remedied with this lifestyle. Even individuals with type 1 diabetes can improve and at least carefully cut down on insulin doses under the care of a practitioner. Once blood sugar is stable and healing has occurred, fasting is then a possibility.

If you decide to incorporate fasting, here's one word of caution. Do not fast one day or one meal and eat double the next. You may be tempted to overeat when you resume eating. Overloading your system with food is not a healthy practice anytime, but especially after fasting.

Fasting has many benefits other than weight loss. You will notice you have more time for other things on fast days, time that would otherwise be consumed by food preparation and eating. Run errands or catch up on other chores. Indulge in the luxury of a nap. Another benefit is a savings in grocery money, money that perhaps you can put toward the extra expense of buying organic foods.

Tell Your Story, Learn from Others

While we encourage you to take a break now and then from eating, you should never stop learning, and you should always keep a journal, two habits that go hand in hand. Together they motivate you to make healthy choices as you try to lose weight or maintain a healthy weight. They also help you hold yourself accountable.

Your journal can be a simple spiral notebook or a fancy cloth-covered journal. In Appendices B and C we offer sample journal pages that you can enlarge, photocopy, and keep in a binder. Using the provided format guides you in what to record; all you have to do is fill it in. The important thing is to keep a record, no matter the method. Take a "before" picture of yourself to put in the front. Record your starting date, weight, all physical symptoms, and emotions. Describe how you feel about your body and your eating habits. As little or as much as you desire may be recorded, but the more you write, the more helpful and encouraging this journal will be later. If you use the forms provided in this book, notebook paper can always be inserted if you need more writing space.

Begin recording all of the food you eat for several days before you start the *NBFA* Lifestyle. This gives you concrete evidence of how you have been eating and suggests the changes you need to make. It also helps you see how much you have changed when you look back later.

Each day you should record the date, the kind of exercise you did, and the length of your workout. Record the hours you slept as well as any unusual stresses. You should also record everything you ate and drank and the time you did so. If you feel particularly bad or good after a meal, jot that down. You will begin to note patterns in how you feel relative to the foods you have consumed. Recording what you eat also helps you to realize how much you are eating, encouraging you to eat less. Record the pH of your first-morning urine, and learn which foods make you too acidic. Be honest and write down all that you eat, or you are only cheating yourself. If you notice difficulty sleeping, problems with elimination, mood swings, headaches, excess mucus, strong cravings, or situations that are very tempting for you, record all of these things. Note all of your triumphs and failures.

Some clients have discovered food allergies or intolerances by noticing symptoms that consistently followed the consumption of certain foods. Over the course of several weeks, Vickie noticed that she had recurring headaches. She recorded them in her journal. She was able to go back and look over what she had eaten prior to the headaches and noticed that each time she experienced headaches she had eaten nuts. You too may discover the sources of certain health problems by noting the correlation between your symptoms and your food patterns.

Andrea was able to track the source of her indigestion by realizing that she experienced difficulty after meals with poor food combinations. At one meal, she ate a vegetarian omelet (vegetables and protein), hash browns (starch), toast with jelly (starch and fruit with processed sugar), and a fruit cup. She broke all the food-combining rules. Some individuals are more sensitive to this than others.

One journal note: We don't encourage you to weigh yourself on a daily basis. It can be too discouraging due to water weight and daily fluctuations. Weigh yourself one day a week and record that weight in your journal. Always weigh on the same day each week. If you are doing some weight training, remember that muscle weighs more than fat. You may notice your clothes are loose even when the scale does not show weight loss. Weekly weigh-ins force you to face reality, positive or negative. Even if you have had a bad week, you need to be honest with yourself. Weighing in can prevent you from getting too far off track.

The sample journal pages also provide space for you to record elimination patterns, water consumption, urine pH, energy level, attitude, exposure to sunlight, and goals. The last thing that should be recorded in your journal are encouraging quotes from your reading or interesting things that you learn. Perhaps you've learned about a positive mind-set, daily physical exercise, nutrition, or a healthy lifestyle. Anything that encourages you should be included.

As you begin to lose weight and gain health, describe how you feel. Note when symptoms diminish or disappear. If you so desire, take new photos of yourself as your results become noticeable. This is going to be a book of encouragement. The more you put into your journal, the more you get out of it. If you are having a hard day, go back and read through the encouragements. If you are tempted to eat something that you know you should not eat, review how you felt the last time you ate that. In this way, your journal becomes a friend and accountability partner.

Be inspired by Paul C. Bragg, often recognized as the founder of America's health movement. Bragg, an author, speaker, and health pioneer, kept a journal for more than seventy years. He enjoyed a long, healthy life that would have continued much longer if not for a tragic accident while surfing in Hawaii in 1976 at the age of ninety-five. He knew the value of journaling and realized it was worth his time to keep a record of his health.

One more important part of the *NBFA* Lifestyle: In working with hundreds of individuals embarking on a new journey of health, we can usually tell who will succeed and who will fail by their desire to learn. Those individuals who realize that learning is unending and who have a passion to keep looking for more information about how to enhance their health usually achieve their goals. People who seem to know it all or who want to be spoon-fed information are not nearly as successful.

Read books, newsletters, magazines, or the Internet. Listen to tapes or CDs, tune in to radio shows, watch DVDs, or attend seminars. Time is a factor for all of us, so you may want to listen to CDs while you exercise or drive, or find other creative ways to increase your learning time. Raymond's website, www. beyondhealth.com, offers a wide array of health information, including articles and access to Raymond's weekly radio show. Raymond also publishes a bimonthly newsletter, *Beyond Health News*. Subscription information is on the website.

Be careful to learn from accurate teachers. Not all of the books and materials available are helpful or health-building. Read what is recommended by authors you trust. You can begin with the list of sources and recommended reading provided in Appendix E. Whatever you read, you must filter it and decide what is true. Many times it just comes down to common sense.

Information feeds your mind and nourishes your motivation. When you are not learning about or reminding yourself that sugar is a deadly poison, you are more likely to succumb to the temptation to eat a donut or pastry. When reading about the benefits of pure drinking water, you are likely to desire to quench your thirst with a glass of water. When reading a chapter on the benefits of juicing, you will likely become eager to make fresh vegetable juice. As you listen to a tape on all of the benefits of exercise, you probably will be motivated to get moving.

If you read something that is particularly helpful, include the thought in your journal. Post motivational quotes on the mirror or by your desk. A list of deadly effects of sugar can be placed on the refrigerator as a daily deterrent. Be like a sponge, ready to absorb all the information you can. Motivational speaker Jim Rohn is known for advising, "Miss a meal, but don't you miss your reading." That is excellent advice.

Putting It into Practice

We have discussed so many new healthy habits that your head is probably full, and you are wondering where to begin. Chapter 12 gives you a plan for easily incorporating this lifestyle into your daily routines—one step at a time. You don't have to master this lifestyle perfectly by tomorrow; you can take it at your own pace. Beginning to move in the right direction is vital. Your body is making hundreds of billions of new cells today. You have the opportunity and the responsibility to optimize the health of these cells. To the extent that you do, you will become younger and healthier.

THE GENETIC PATHWAY

I n this chapter you learn about the role of genetics in your health and weight and discover how to manage the expression of the genes you inherited. This chapter provides insight into:

- How wrong food choices turn on fat-storing genes.
- Why overweight seems to run in families.
- Changes you can make to optimize the expression of your genes and live a disease-free, fat-free life.

Nutrition can alter the course of high-risk genes, not only by turning these genes off but also by inhibiting the resulting bad effects produced by them.

—Russell L. Blaylock
Health and Nutrition Secrets

By the time Diana sought Raymond's help, she weighed three hundred pounds. She had tried nearly every weight-loss diet and gimmick she could find, but she always failed. Because Diana's family members were also obese, she concluded that being fat was her destiny—programmed deep inside her genetic makeup and something over which she had no control. Her conclusion was a sad and dangerous one, and far too common—even among doctors. And her conclusion was wrong.

A strictly genetic cause for overweight, one that cannot be altered with diet and exercise, does happen, but it is very rare. Genes do play an important role in how our bodies store fat, but what we eat and how we live are the determining factors in whether these genes are turned "on" or "off" and how they manifest. The key to permanent weight loss is to keep your fat-burning genes turned on and your fat-storing genes turned off. If you do this, you lose weight automatically. Poor eating habits, toxic exposures, and unhealthy lifestyles shared by family members are more often the reason that obesity appears to be inherited. That was true for Diana. Following the *NBFA* Lifestyle, she lost 120 pounds in the first fifteen months. She feels immensely better and more energized, and she suffers far fewer of the numerous health problems she suffered before, including frequent colds. By eating nutritious whole foods, taking high-quality supplements, avoiding toxins, and exercising, Diana's genes got the message: stop storing fat.

Recent research gives us a whole new understanding of genes, the role they play in human health, and how each of us has the power to control what happens. Genes are important to everything that happens in the body, yet the average person has little understanding of what genes are and even less understanding of what controls them. A gene is a sequence of DNA that determines an inherited characteristic. This unit of inheritance is copied and transmitted from one generation to the next. Genes determine factors such as our eye color and hair color, but diet and lifestyle have tremendous impact on how our genes establish our size and shape. At least several genes appear to have the ability to affect weight control, but none of these genes seems to play the lead role in determining how much we weigh. The lead role is played by the instructions that we give those genes. If we don't like the results, we need to change the instructions. Scientific breakthroughs in our understanding of how genes interact with nutrients and toxins to turn them on or off give us the tools we need to control weight permanently.

Wrong Diet Can Turn On "Fat" Genes

Although we tend to think of genes as unchangeable, such as the genes that control the color of our eyes or our hair, most genes are far more flexible. Think of them as obedient servants, changing how they express from day to day and even minute to minute, depending on the instructions you give them. Furthermore, just because a gene is present does not mean that specific trait is going to manifest. A pea plant with a genetic tendency toward tallness will not achieve its full size if it is deprived of adequate water and minerals required for optimal growth. Himalayan rabbits, whose native climate is cold, have genes that give them black ears, forepaws, noses, and tails, but if these rabbits are raised in warm temperatures, those black markings do not appear.

Genes, therefore, activate only under certain environmental conditions. Far from being a sure-fire determinant that something will happen, genes are a potential for something to happen. All of us have genetic predispositions, such as to gum disease, Parkinson's disease, Crohn's disease, insulin resistance, cancer, or overweight. Genes have the potential to invite that disease or encourage overweight, but what you do with your life almost always tells the final story. Genes may run our lives, but we run the genes—so we run our lives!

Understanding the true nature of genes gives you the power over disease. You turn genes on and off through the chemical, physical, electromagnetic, and mental environments you create. Your diet is critical. Nutrient-rich foods create a chemical environment in each cell that keeps the health-producing genes turned on and the fat-storing, disease-producing, and rapid-aging genes turned off, which is why diseases can be both prevented and reversed by what you eat. Chronic diseases, including cancer, heart disease, type 2 diabetes, and overweight, are all known to be reversible with optimal nutrition. Beyond diet, avoiding environmental chemicals that can alter the expression of our genes is also critical. If you eat an excellent diet, avoid toxins, get exercise, and control stress, you can enjoy a very long and disease-free life, just as long-lived populations in other parts of the world have done in the past.

Some of the signals that influence genetic behavior come from hormone activity. Eating sugar and refined carbohydrates, ingredients that are so prevalent in processed food, increases your insulin level and disrupts your hormone balance. Out-of-whack hormones send the wrong instructions to your genes, telling them to store fat. Even worse, those same signals turn on genes that contribute to aging and to other illnesses.

In addition to the effects of the hormones produced in our bodies, we are exposed to hormones when we eat most meat and dairy products, which disrupts our hormone balance and sends inappropriate signals to genes.

Another concern is the evidence that certain environmental toxins disrupt our hormones and send erroneous signals to our genes, even blocking legitimate signals. Since hormones are part of our endocrine system, the hormone disrupters are called endocrine disrupters. Toxic chemicals such as certain pesticides and herbicides, dioxins, PCBs, phthalates, and bisphenol A are all capable of acting as endocrine disrupters and sending signals to genes that can result in fat storage. A major source of these toxins is conventional meat and dairy products.

You May Have Inherited Your Overweight Habits

Throughout human history, finding adequate amounts of food on a regular basis was seldom assured. Our ancestors' bodies stored any excess food as fat, and then used that fat as a fuel source, working it off when food was scarce. Many of us—estimated at 85 percent of the population—have a biological makeup that is very efficient at storing fat. When food is plentiful, rather than scarce, what used to be a biological advantage tips the scales in the wrong direction. Many of us live in societies in which excess food is almost always available, particularly fattening, nutrient-poor junk food. Our biological efficiency at storing fat is now working against us, and if we continue eating too much, we continue to store fat.

Our unique mechanisms to cope with food scarcity, which took a long time to develop, have not adapted to the opposite—chronic overabundance of food. The problem is made worse by the fact that our abundant food supply consists mostly of unhealthy food. Children born to obese parents often have a lower resting metabolism rate, which makes them more susceptible to weight gain. But genes alone do not and cannot explain the explosion in overweight disease over the last several decades. Our diet and lifestyle are to blame. We consume too much calorie-loaded sugar, white flour, fat, soda, and alcohol; we consume more calories than we burn, are exposed to too many toxins, and are physically inactive. *The environmental provocation of excess calories, toxicity, and physical inactivity is necessary to make overweight happen on the massive scale we are experiencing.*

To take a look at real-life examples of the roles that genes do and do not play in weight control, we can look to the experiences of the Pima Indian tribe of Mexico. The Pima Indians developed superior fat-storing survival skills to sustain them through periods of food scarcity. As we have talked about before, this kind of genetic survival tool is an advantage when food is scarce, but a problem—a susceptibility to weight gain—when food is plentiful. Part of the Pima tribe lives in Mexico. Those people tend to work hard and eat a traditional low-calorie, nutrient-rich, whole-food diet consisting of staples such as beans, corn, and potatoes, along with fresh seasonal fruits and vegetables. Other tribe members live across the border in Arizona. These Pimas have adopted a typical American, high-calorie, low-nutrient, junk-food diet and a sedentary lifestyle. The result: The Mexican Pimas are healthy, slim, and fit. The American Pimas are obese and sick, suffering the world's highest rate of obesity and type 2 diabetes—same ancestors, same genes, different diets and lifestyle, and dramatically different results. *Genes play a role, but diet and lifestyle are the determining factors.* By eating a diet rich in nutrients and fiber, while low in toxins, and remaining physically active, the Mexican Pimas maintained good health and normal weight by giving their fat-control genes the correct instructions.

To optimize your health and weight on the Genetic Pathway, eat and live in harmony with your genes: Do not eat toxic processed foods; eat organic whole foods that are automatically nutrient-rich, low-calorie, and toxin-free; take high-quality supplements; reduce stress; and get regular exercise, sunlight, and proper rest. Create a positive, uplifting environment for your cells, and your genes will get the message and act accordingly. You will be healthy, slim, and vigorous, and live to a very old age free of disease and disability.

THE MEDICAL **10** PATHWAY

Buyer Beware

In this chapter you learn why you need to take personal charge of your wellness and weight-loss plans and not depend upon solutions from conventional medicine with its prescriptions and surgical procedures. In fact, you'll discover how little your doctor may know and how blindly accepting what he or she prescribes could be dangerous. This chapter highlights:

- How weight-loss drugs sabotage health.
- Why liposuction and gastric bypass surgeries are not good choices.
- Why prescription drugs and medical care can be deadly.
- Why current medical practices are obsolete.

- The startling lack of nutrition education required for medical doctors.
- Why taking personal responsibility for your health is so important.

The modern medical paradigm is stuck at the turn of the century. . . . Lacking a paradigm broad and deep enough to enable scientists and practitioners to progress, medicine is in many ways paralyzed.

—Joseph D. Beasley
The Kellogg Report (1989)

Because overweight is a disease, you might be compelled to look for answers at your doctor's office. To that, we would say: Caution When Entering. Modern medicine, as it is commonly practiced, does nothing to address the true causes of disease, and more often than not, doctors and the drugs they prescribe make you sicker and fatter. Modern mainstream medical science is not your answer to optimal health or permanent weight control.

Moving toward health and weight control on the Medical Pathway requires knowledge and caution. Only a limited number of cutting-edge physicians and other practitioners can lead you in the right direction, one that sustains you throughout your life. Most physicians have a limited set of tools that they offer the sick: drugs, radiation, and surgery. Desperate people often turn to drugs and surgeries in an effort to lose weight, yet these outmoded treatments have proven themselves to be both ineffective and dangerous.

The major reason modern medicine (also known as allopathic medicine or conventional medicine) is ineffective in treating overweight and obesity is the same reason it is ineffective in treating any chronic disease: *modern medicine treats the symptoms of disease but does nothing to correct the underlying causes.* Physicians use powerful synthetic chemicals to suppress symptoms and keep the patient out of immediate danger, while the patient continues the unhealthy lifestyle that caused the problem in the first place. Traditional physicians have been inadequately educated within a system that clings to outdated thinking. Most physicians are simply unaware of the awesome scientific advances that have occurred over the last century and particularly over the last few decades. Deficiency and toxicity are the two causes of disease, yet the overwhelming majority of physicians have little or no understanding of this. Nutrition may be the single most important factor in preventing and reversing disease and overweight, yet most physicians have virtually no training in nutrition and assume that the vast majority of illnesses have no connection to nutrition. When is the last time—if this ever happened—that your doctor asked you in detail about your nutrition? Have you and your doctor ever had a serious and detailed discussion about vitamins and minerals? Has your doctor ever asked about your exposure to common toxins? Is there time during your office visit when you are asked about the emotional stresses in your life? How strongly does your physician insist upon regular exercise and fresh air as part of your prescription for health? When was the last time your doctor suggested that you could choose how your genes are expressed by the way that you live? Without recognizing the true causes of disease and overweight, physicians are reduced to merely managing symptoms by writing costly prescriptions for toxic chemicals and doing unnecessary surgery. Diseases and obesity remain chronic, patients suffer, and medical and social costs continue to increase.

Conventional doctors look at the body one organ at a time without developing an understanding of the body as a whole, which is critical to holistic health—the only true state of health. When one part of the body malfunctions, that part is singled out by conventional medicine and its many specialists. Disease is seen as confined to specific locations or organs, rather than affecting the whole person. But disease happens because cells malfunction, causing the body's self-regulating and balancing mechanisms to malfunction, which affects the entire body, not just one part. When you are sick, you are sick all over. Conventional doctors try to force disease into submission through drugs and surgery, which only throw the body further out of balance. Today's doctors are taught that "cures" come from outside the body, while the truth is that the human body has a natural capacity to heal itself. The focus should be on that natural healing process and on giving your body what it needs to do its job. That is why the *NBFA* Lifestyle focuses on cellular health; the whole body is made of cells. Problems at the cellular level cause overweight disease. In order to achieve permanent weight loss, you must pay attention to all Six Pathways along which healthy cells are supported. Once your cells are healthy, disease and excess weight simply vanish.

The Dangers of Diet Drugs, Liposuction, and Gastric Bypass

A variety of drugs have been used to try to treat obesity, but no magic pill exists. Some weight-loss drugs are designed to increase the levels of certain brain chemicals in order to suppress appetite. Other "diet" drugs are intended to inhibit fat metabolism in the gut, causing less fat to be absorbed. Still other weight-loss drugs have proven to be so dangerous—causing heart-valve problems, for example—that they are no longer used, while many have just failed in their mission. On average, people on these drugs lose only 5 to 10 percent of their original weight. If you start at three hundred pounds, you may lose only fifteen to thirty pounds—hardly a victory. The success rate of weight-reduction drugs is minimal, and what little success there is comes at a high price; side effects are numerous and can be dangerous.

One popular weight-control drug is Xenical. Xenical works by blocking fat from being absorbed, but its benefits are marginal, and it has tremendous side effects. It can cause significant hormonal and nutritional imbalances, including the loss of critical fat-soluble vitamin absorption. And if you eat fat, it can cause severe stomach pain and uncontrollable diarrhea. (The manufacturer is now planning an over-the-counter version of Xenical called Alli.) Some consumers are so shortsighted and anxious to drop pounds that they do anything for the immediate gratification of weight loss and choose not to consider the long-term problems that these risky drugs may initiate.

Doctors usually recommend that weight-control drugs be used in conjunction with a healthy diet and regular exercise, but a healthy diet and regular exercise by themselves reduce weight—no drugs required. The drugs merely take credit for benefits derived from improvements in eating and lifestyle. Doctors also prescribe numerous drugs to treat the complications of obesity, including cholesterol, diabetes, and blood-pressure medications. These, too, come with long lists of health-damaging side effects. Worse still, such medications can actually make you gain weight as certain drugs and combinations of drugs interfere with the body's water management, appetite, and weight-control systems.

A common option offered to overweight people is liposuction, a surgical procedure during which fat is literally sucked out. Liposuction results in weight loss, at least temporarily, but this procedure is not benign and comes with an assortment of dangerous side effects, including infections and even death.

The death rate for liposuction is twenty times higher than for other elective surgery.

Gastric bypass surgery (bariatric surgery) creates a much smaller stomach by removing part of the stomach. This procedure makes you feel full faster, and you learn to reduce the amount of food that you eat at any given time. The small intestine is rearranged and attached to the new stomach. In April 2005, an article in *USA Today* reported that gastric bypass surgery is by far "the most effective option for severely obese people." Let's see if you agree. This surgery does help people to lose some weight (an average of only fifty-five pounds), but gastric bypass surgery does absolutely nothing to address the causes of obesity, and it comes with some extremely dangerous side effects, including malnutrition, infection, digestive problems, and death. What really happens is they rip out part of your digestive system, staple you back together, and call it a "weight-loss plan." Overweight people are already malnourished, and to create more malnourishment by causing you to eat less is catastrophic to health. Even if you try to eat a healthy diet, you will not get or absorb enough nutrition. Nonetheless, the popularity of bariatric surgery has exploded, up 400 percent between 1998 and 2002. By far the largest increase was for patients between the ages of fifty-five and sixty-four, a 900 percent increase for that age group. The annual cost of these surgeries is now $5 billion and increasing rapidly.

While costly, gastric bypass surgery is only marginally effective, and the risk of complications is virtually 100 percent, including a high risk of death. The *Journal of the American Medical Association* reported in October 2005 that the death rate for men aged thirty-five to forty-four was more than 5 percent, and that the rate among sixty-five- to seventy-year-olds was 13 percent. In patients older than seventy-five, half of the patients who opted for this surgery died! In 2005, 145,000 of these surgeries were performed, and 1,400 of these people died right on the operating table.

Severe hypoglycemia (low blood sugar) is one dangerous side effect of bariatric surgery. Some patients become confused and lightheaded and experience rapid heartbeats. Many shake, sweat, and suffer headaches. Some patients even fall unconscious due to low blood sugar, which has been linked to a number of auto accidents. Internal hernias, a devastating postoperative complication that leads to intestinal obstruction, also can occur long after surgery. There is also an increased risk of blood clots, which continues beyond the immediate postoperative period. The main risk, though, is pulmonary embolism (a blood clot in the lungs) that can occur up to two years after the surgery. Physicians often prescribe blood thinners to avoid such clots, but this increases the risk of bleeding so that internal hemorrhage is both a common and alarming side effect. Even under the best of circumstances, surgery-related complications may continue for a lifetime and are often life-threatening. Too often the resulting weight loss is only temporary. Some people, for the love of food, have managed to stretch their surgically undersized stomachs and put the weight back on. They never learned to change their lifestyle, and the result is temporary change only. The *NBFA* Lifestyle is a safe and far more effective option, offering lifetime success to even morbidly obese individuals.

Modern medicine's latest weapon for fighting fat is a European development—inserting a balloon into the stomach to make the stomach feel full and to reduce food consumption for a period of time. In this procedure, a balloon is inserted down the patient's throat and into the stomach where it is filled with a saline solution. The balloon is removed after six months. This is just another nonsensical approach to weight control. It does not address why the patient is overweight, and as such, patients can expect to regain their weight after the balloon is gone. Further, this procedure also has risks and side effects.

Medical education continues to be wedded to outmoded models, with our physicians poorly educated in nutrition, biochemistry, physiology, and biophysics. Most medical education is directed toward pharmaceutical drugs, which cure nothing and, worse, do harm—all of which points to why we need to educate ourselves and take personal responsibility for our health.

SUPPLEMENTS ARE ESSENTIAL

S ince overweight is primarily a nutritional deficiency disease, supplements can help give cells what they need, shutting off the appetite. High-quality food and supplements can also help to supply your detoxification system with the raw materials it needs to detoxify chemicals that jam your appetite and fat-storing controls. Tragically, most supplements are junk! Read on for help to sort through the junk and find what is worthwhile. In this chapter, you will learn:

- Which nutrients are most essential.
- How prescription drugs can deplete nutrients.
- The possible results of even one nutrient deficiency.
- Suggestions for choosing from among the many supplements.
- Cheap ingredients to avoid.

- Why the manufacturing, storage, and shipping processes for supplements are so important.
- Details on three critical vitamins—C, E, and D.

The nutritional microenvironment of our body cells is crucially important to our health and . . . deficiencies in this environment constitute a major cause of disease.

—Roger J. Williams
Nutrition Against Disease

Diet pills? Don't even think about it. But if you want your weight loss to be successful and permanent, you should include something else in pill form: essential vitamins, minerals, and other nutrients taken as supplements.

One of the biggest fallacies today is the myth that you can get all the nutrients you need for good health and long life by eating a so-called balanced diet. Given the reality of today's nutritionally depleted foods, this is next to impossible, which is why you must fill in the gaps by supplementing those missing nutrients. If you do not, those gaps sabotage your body's biochemical balance, stimulate your appetite, keep you hungry, encourage unwanted pounds, and undermine your best efforts to stay trim.

You may already agree that multivitamins are a good idea. In fact, you may have been taking a multivitamin for years, but you may not understand the full picture. Perhaps you have never considered vitamins and minerals to be weight-loss aids because you don't understand the role they play in your body's functions. Furthermore, most people don't know how to choose supplements that work. If you choose low-quality products, no matter what they cost, despite your good intentions they will not help you to lose weight and to stay healthy.

The materials and methods used to make supplements determine whether they are helpful, almost useless, or even harmful. This chapter helps you find your way through the maze of supplement products on the market today. There is no way for you to know how a product is manufactured, stored, shipped, and distributed simply by looking at the product, its advertisement, or even its label. You need expert advice. You can educate yourself, however, about the different forms in which vitamins and minerals are manufactured and how to recognize the most beneficial types on your own, including how to recognize indicators of quality on product labels.

To help you get well, stay well, and lose weight, this chapter offers a primer on vitamins, your basic ABCs—from vitamin A to the B vitamins to vitamin C, and beyond. You should understand which vitamins and minerals are responsible for which functions and how a deficiency can result in disease and overweight. Further—and few people possess this information—you should learn how vitamins, minerals, and other nutrients interact with and depend on each other. Without that information, you could undermine your hard work to stay healthy and lose weight.

Once you learn this and make wise purchases, each day's task becomes simple: take the supplements you need, and your weight and health will respond. Your body knows what to do. You just need to make sure you give your body the essential raw materials. What should you take each day? As a minimum, we recommend that most people take at least a multivitamin/mineral formula, extra vitamin C, and essential fatty acids every day. Beyond that, we recommend vitamin E, bioflavonoids, calcium, and magnesium. (You learn more about all of these later in this chapter.) Anyone with an active disease needs additional vitamin C and other nutrients tailored to his or her specific cellular deficiencies. If you are overweight, supplement with antioxidants including vitamins C and E to protect yourself from free-radical oxidative damage. Because fat cells produce a flood of free radicals, these radicals must be neutralized by antioxidants, or they will age your tissues and damage your DNA, causing mutations.

Don't be misled, though. Supplements cannot do the job by themselves. By now you understand that in order to stay healthy you must eat a diet of fresh, whole foods full of nutrients in the right balance.

Feed Your Cells Well

A living cell is enormously complex. Think of each one of your tens of trillions of microscopic cells as a vast industrial park containing thousands of factories, hundreds of powerhouses, warehouses, distribution centers, raw material delivery systems, waste disposal systems, internal and external communications systems, security systems, and much more. Each of these industrial parks creates a vast array of products that are necessary to keep you alive and well, including neurotransmitters for your nervous system, high-energy compounds to power your metabolic machinery, antibodies for your immune system, and hormones for your endocrine system.

More than one hundred thousand critical chemical reactions take place in each cell every second, each requiring what in an industrial factory would be called raw materials. In our bodies, these raw materials are called nutrients. In a factory, a chronic lack of even one raw material impairs the ability to make products. The same is true for the body; a chronic lack of even one nutrient causes cellular malfunction and disease.

Given the complex needs of our cell factories, how is the average American doing regarding nutrition? According to the USDA's 1996 Continuing Survey of Food Intakes, not very well. More than 70 percent of Americans do not consume the recommended daily allowance for zinc. Eighty percent do not get enough vitamin B_6, and 75 percent do not get sufficient magnesium. Other common nutrient deficiencies include vitamins A, B_1, B_2, B_{12}, C, and D, and calcium, iron, enzymes, and essential fatty acids.

Depleted soils, resulting from intensive farming, the use of artificial fertilizers, and poor crop rotation practices plus premature harvesting, long transit times to market, processing, and a host of other factors have *drastically* reduced the nutritional quality of our food. The average American gets only a fraction of the nutrition they need for optimal health, but most people are totally unaware of this. They think that the produce they buy at the supermarket is of the same quality as what our ancestors ate. Not so. For example, in 2001 a study in *The Nutrition Practitioner,* a peer-reviewed scientific journal, looked at calcium levels in food over the period 1940–1991. On average, in the space of fifty years, the calcium content of vegetables dropped by 46 percent. You can be sure it is even lower today. In short, you have to eat twice as much broccoli today to get the same amount of calcium that people were getting in 1940. Similarly, magnesium in fresh produce has been reduced by an average of 24 percent. All bodily processes depend on the action and interaction of minerals. A shortage of even one can throw the entire body out of balance. As Nobel Prize–winner Dr. Linus Pauling once said, "You can trace every sickness, every disease, and every ailment to a mineral deficiency." The 1992 Earth Summit Report suggests that 99 percent of Americans are mineral deficient. No wonder so many of us are sick and overweight.

Not only are our soils deficient in minerals, but also critical mineral ratios have been disturbed so that we no longer get a proper balance of minerals. Minerals rely on being present in specific relationships with other nutrients. For example, the body wants twice as much calcium as phosphorous. Modern farming has disturbed these critical ratios. In the last 50 years, fresh carrots have lost 75 percent of their magnesium, 48 percent of their calcium, 46 percent of their iron, and 75 percent of their copper, with similar kinds of losses for other vegetables. These losses throw the natural mineral ratios out of balance. These imbalances would appear even greater if we were to compare current levels with levels in the food available one hundred years ago. Current studies on "fresh" oranges have found that many contain no vitamin C whatsoever!

It's bad enough that our modern food lacks nutrients, but we further deplete what little nutrition we get from our diet. One of those agents of depletion is prescription drugs, which are taken by half the American population. Medications cause nutritional deficiencies by lowering blood levels of critical vitamins and minerals. For example, millions of people take cholesterol-lowering drugs, but these drugs deplete crucial nutrients such as coenzyme Q_{10} as well as vitamins and minerals such as A, B_{12}, D, E, calcium, magnesium, and zinc. Although we hope you can avoid prescription drugs, if you do take them it is important to research how those drugs affect nutrients so that you can supplement your diet accordingly. This is information your doctor may not tell you—information he or she may not even know.

Malnutrition Despite Our Abundance

It has been estimated that our distant ancestors consumed three to four times more nutrients than we get today, *yet the changes in our environment and lifestyle make our need for nutrients higher than ever.* Due to the abundance of toxins in our environment, more raw materials are required to help our bodies cope with incoming toxins and to rid our systems of accumulated toxins. For instance, the chlorine in our water, ozone in our air, and many other environmental pollutants create an oxidizing environment that requires massive amounts of antioxidants to neutralize. Unless we supply our bodies with massive amounts of antioxidants, oxidative free-radical damage will occur, DNA will be damaged, and we will get older and sicker. Meanwhile, our stressful lifestyles require large quantities of nutrients. The very manufacturing of stress chemicals depletes precious vitamins and minerals. Given that a shortage of even one nutrient will cause disease, we would have to eat an extraordinarily nutritious diet to meet this historically unprecedented need for nutrients. So are we eating an extraordinary diet? Yes, we are—*one that is extraordinarily deficient in essential nutrients.* The typical low-quality food we get at supermarkets and restaurants is not the kind of fresh, whole, living food that supplies our cells with all the nutrients they need to provide us with good health. Unfortunately, modern medicine all but ignores these realities.

Most people are unaware of the unprecedented burden that our exposure to toxins is placing on our bodies, dramatically increasing our need for nutrients, particularly antioxidants. Indeed, studies have shown that our need for antioxidants has *tripled* since 1970. Meanwhile the antioxidant level in foods has been *cut in half*! When you consider that the need in 1970 was already greatly elevated over historical levels, you can begin to understand that the declining nutritional content of our foods and our increased nutritional needs are a prescription for an epidemic of malnutrition, disease, and overweight. The bottom line is this: the need for nutrients is up while the supply is down. Supplements are necessary to bridge the gap.

Feeling Tired? Check Your Nutrients

Most people are familiar with the term Recommended Dietary Allowances (RDA), which is now part of something more comprehensive called the Dietary Reference Intakes (DRI). RDAs are those levels of vitamins and minerals that the Food and Nutrition Board of the National Academy of Sciences has established as guidelines to prevent the kind of nutrient deficiencies that lead to obvious deficiency diseases such as scurvy (vitamin C deficiency), pellagra (vitamin B_3 deficiency), and beriberi (vitamin B_1 deficiency). The RDA is not the amount required to achieve optimal health. The RDA is only what is required to prevent obvious deficiency disease in most people; the amount required to optimize health is much higher. Even though the RDA is less than what is needed for optimal health, very few of us are getting the RDA for all of our nutrients on a regular basis. Even small shortages of nutrients result in subclinical deficiencies (before recognizable symptoms are observed). Subclinical deficiencies lead to less obvious, though often no less serious, disease states. All of us have days when we don't quite feel like ourselves. We might be a little tired or achy, or have a pain here or there. But when we often experience muscle aches and pains of no known origin or have frequent colds or other infections, nutritional deficiencies are usually the cause. Subclinical deficiencies, usually the result of a flawed diet, can weaken the immune system, cause colds and flu, and lead to various chronic disease states depending on which nutrient is lacking.

Subclinical deficiencies can be insidious because it is hard to know we have them. This is why such deficiencies now affect virtually everyone. Chronic diseases such as heart disease, high blood pressure, and cancer are known to be more prevalent in people who consume fewer nutrient-rich fresh fruits, vegetables, high-fiber grains, and legumes. Fortunately, such deficiencies can be corrected with diet, supplements, and lifestyle modification.

A nutrient deficiency may also result from your unique biochemistry. Each of us is biologically unique ("biochemical individuality"). Each of us has a unique need for nutrients and an above-average need for one or more nutrients. In fact, one person may need as much as forty times more of a particular nutrient than another person. Thus, two people eating the same diet may achieve different results. One may be adequately provisioned and healthy, while the other is deficient and sick. For example, at least one-third of all cases of schizophrenia result from higher-than-ordinary needs for minerals such as zinc and vitamins such as B_3, B_6, B_{12}, and folic acid. Rather than being medicated or hospitalized, these patients can recover completely when their above-average nutritional needs are met. There is no such thing as an RDA that applies to everyone.

Unfortunately, there is no practical way to measure how much of each vitamin and mineral your body really needs, which is why we must always strive for optimal nutrition. We cannot afford to eat junk foods that are loaded with calories and empty of nutrition. It is also why it is critical that we eat a wide variety of living foods loaded with nutrients. Although RDA guidelines reflect average requirements, most Americans are not even getting the RDA. How could they when close to a third of the average person's caloric intake comes from sugar, white flour, sodas, and other empty-calorie junk foods?

Supplements Are Essential, but Many Products Are Useless

In June 2002, a landmark study published in the *Journal of the American Medical Association,* analyzing thirty-six years of data, concluded that *everyone needs a daily multivitamin regardless of age or health.* Four years earlier, in April 1998, the National Academy of Sciences issued a profound statement saying that most people will not get all the vitamins they need even if they eat a good diet with lots of fruits and vegetables. In our modern world, *supplementing is essential.*

Many Americans take notice of the need for supplements, but their choices lead them down unhealthy paths and dead ends. Although Americans spend almost $20 billion on supplements every year, they are getting sicker and fatter. You may have heard people say that all you really get from taking vitamins is expensive urine. Lending credence to this view, large-scale epidemiological studies by the federal Centers for Disease Control and the National Research Council (NRC) have failed to find any health benefits among people who take vitamins. In July 2002, an Oxford University study published in the medical journal *Lancet* announced that vitamins are "a waste of money." Other studies have found specific vitamins such as vitamins C, E, and beta carotene to be ineffective and, at times, dangerous.

These findings fly in the face of decades of work and thousands of scientific studies showing the benefits of vitamins. So which side is right? They both are! Supplements are beneficial, but most vitamin supplement products are not of sufficient quality to measure benefits. A sad fact: *Most of the money spent these days on supplements is wasted because most supplements are not worth what you pay for them.*

It is important to learn how to select and take supplement products that *are* worth your money, but supplements are *not* a substitute for real food. Nothing can replace the nutrition provided by living foods. For example, a tomato contains thousands of different chemicals. We have no idea how many of those are necessary to human health or how they all work together. Try duplicating that in a pill!

Many people take multivitamins hoping to compensate for their poor diets. Advertisements cater to these misplaced hopes, but simply supplementing a poor diet can never lead to good health. It would be preferable if we could get all of our vitamins and minerals from nutritious food, as our ancestors did, but the quality of the modern food supply is too low. If we hope to thrive in today's world, we must optimize our diets *and* take high-quality supplements.

How to Find High-Quality Supplements

How do you find safe and effective supplement products? As it turns out, this task is not easy. Poor formulation, adulteration, substandard manufacturing practices, and substitution of inferior ingredients are rampant in this industry. You can get a sense of how difficult it is from a landmark study reported in the winter 1999 *Journal of the American Nutraceutical Association*. This study found that only 2.5 percent of the commonly available nutritional products studied were both nontoxic and effective. In other words, 97.5 percent of supplements they studied were either toxic and/or ineffective.

Many thousands of vitamin brands are sold, but few are effective. New supplement products come out almost weekly, often making outlandish claims, but few are worth what you pay for them. The cheapest brands are usually the worst bargains because they provide little to no benefit, and they are usually loaded with cheap fillers and contaminated with solvent residues, artificial food colors and flavors, allergens, and other potentially harmful chemicals. Unfortunately, even many higher-priced brands provide little benefit. Too many companies spend their money on advertising, not on creating a quality product that will synergize with the body's biochemical pathways and provide the most nutrition. Quality ingredients are expensive. Even if quality ingredients are used, proper care in the manufacturing process can make a huge difference in the final product. Temperature, humidity, exposure to light, processing time, and other factors must be carefully controlled. Offers in the mail or at drugstores and supermarkets for cut-rate vitamins are virtually always a poor choice.

The scientific literature assumes that the body utilizes between 5 and 25 percent of a vitamin or mineral supplement, but properly formulated high-quality supplements can achieve far higher utilization rates. However, even this 5 to 25 percent assumption is based on another assumption: that digestion is perfect and that all of the necessary transporters, protectors, and enablers are present to properly metabolize the nutrients. Unfortunately, these assumptions are not valid for most Americans. Three out of four Americans have a diagnosable chronic disease; their metabolism is compromised, making them unable to utilize nutrients at the assumed rate of 5 to 25 percent. Many supplement formulas contain something close to the RDA, but if you are metabolizing less than 5 percent of what is in the pill, you will not come near to supplying what you need by taking such a low-potency formula. This is another reason why it is so difficult to measure any benefits resulting from vitamin consumption.

One reason for the low utilization of nutrients from supplements is that metabolizing these nutrients requires energy. Most supplement formulations assume this energy is available, but in those whose health is compromised, energy deficits are common. The number-one complaint made to doctors is fatigue or lack of energy. When cells lack energy, nutrient uptake is impaired. One way to get around this is to supply energizing factors in the supplement itself. Adding energizing factors (nutrients that help cells produce energy) substantially increases nutrient intake, but it costs more, so few supplement manufacturers do it.

Most vitamins on the market today are synthetics, which often contain toxins and exhibit low biological activity. As an alternative to synthetics, some supplement manufacturers offer products that have been extracted from fresh fruits and vegetables. On the surface this appears to make sense, but unfortunately it doesn't work well in practice. Such extracts rarely retain the biological activity of natural foods. Most deliver only a small quantity of nutrients and are deficient in key nutrients because they undergo extensive nutrient losses due to oxidation and heat-related damage. For example, the vitamin B_{12} in these products has been transformed from a biologically active form into one that is useless. Often touted as "superfoods," they come nowhere near the hype.

Another trend, often accompanied by big marketing hype, is for processed food manufacturers to fortify their products with vitamins and minerals to make them more attractive to the buyer, but these products almost always contain cheap, poorly formulated, biologically inappropriate vitamins and minerals. The minerals are in inorganic forms such as calcium carbonate and magnesium oxide, which have low bioavailability. The vitamins are no better. I often see beverage products that are supplemented with B vitamins sitting under bright lights in the refrigerated section, and the light is actively destroying any little good that these cheap vitamins may have done. Don't fool yourself into thinking that breakfast cereals and other processed foods are any better for you because they are fortified with junk vitamins and minerals.

Some supplement manufacturers try to awe you with the fifty or sixty ingredients they put in their product, but the amount of each is usually too small to be of therapeutic value. Often such products list certain nutrients on the label only to impress the buyer, but when you examine the amount, it is minuscule. For example, one popular antioxidant formula lists alpha-lipoic acid, a valuable antioxidant. Seeing this on the label reassures the buyer, but the problem is it contains only *100 micrograms*—an amount so small that it is worthless. The formula would need to contain at least one thousand times that much to be of value.

Choosing good products is a task for an expert. It takes a vast amount of knowledge, care, and expense to create an effective supplement. The quality of the raw materials used to create almost any product largely determines the quality of the finished product. Biologically, it is no different. The quality of the nutrients used in your supplement has a big influence on how they are used in your body and the effect they have on your health. Any particular vitamin or mineral can have a vastly different biological effect depending on its chemical form, purity, and quality. Since the basis of competition in the supplement market is price, companies have little incentive to spend the money to create quality. The buyer cannot see the quality, and without knowing a lot of chemistry, cannot understand the differences. Reading labels almost never gives sufficient information to fully evaluate a supplement. In fact, two identical labels can represent two vastly different products. You have to understand what is going on behind the label. There are only a few dozen scientists in the United States today who truly understand how to create an effective supplement, and their expertise comes at a price. Add to that the cost of high-quality ingredients and optimal manufacturing, storage, and shipping practices. Then factor in the time and money it would take to educate the consumer as to why your product is better, and you can see why very few manufacturers even attempt to make and market a high-quality supplement.

Supplement Buyer Beware

Poor-quality supplements suffer from several other problems, including their resistance to being effectively dissolved once ingested and their inclusion of allergens and other problematic ingredients. Studies have shown that almost half of all vitamin formulas do not dissolve soon enough to be absorbed by the body. Binders, used to hold the pill together, can prevent it from dissolving. Inexpensive brands are the worst offenders. Never take time-release vitamins; they are coated to prevent their being dissolved until they reach a certain point in the digestive system. Unfortunately, they often pass this point before being dissolved. Lubricants, used to improve flow in the manufacturing process, can also bind tightly to the nutrient particles and prevent them from being dissolved. High-quality binders and lubricants can be used, but it is more expensive to use them. The particle size of the powder also makes a difference in how fast the nutrients will dissolve; finer sizes dissolve faster but cost more and are more difficult to handle.

Almost all vitamins on the market are synthetic, made from petroleum-based chemicals. Unfortunately, synthetic vitamins can be fundamentally different from vitamins found in nature. Quality products are derived from natural molecules and are obtainable, but they cost more. Petroleum-based synthetics lack the natural cofactor and synergist molecules found in food. The most serious problem is the shape of their molecules, which are often the mirror image of their natural counterparts. The analogy is similar to comparing your right hand to your left hand; both hands are the same—yet fundamentally different. It is the precise shape of a molecule that tells the body what to do with it. For example, synthetic beta-carotene is a 100 percent left-handed molecule, while natural beta-carotene is mostly right-handed, which is why synthetic carotene is a poor choice; it has the wrong shape, and studies have shown it to be *unhelpful*. A slightly different shape will produce different results, often with ineffective or even toxic outcomes. Synthetic vitamin E is not well absorbed and less biologically active than natural vitamin E. Further, synthetic vitamin E can interfere with the absorption of beta-carotene from our food and lower carotene levels in the blood. Synthetic vitamin E acetate should never be taken. It has very little antioxidant and anticancer effects and can cause the loss of carotenes from the liver.

Many supplement ingredients are derived from food sources, but the cheapest sources of those are also common allergens, such as corn, milk, wheat, and soy. It costs more to use less allergenic sources. Unfortunately, information regarding the source is not listed on the label. Usually when a label claims to be allergen-free, it means that the ingredients are made from petrochemicals. However, even in such formulas, additives such as the fillers, binders, and lubricants often contain allergens. Taking a vitamin product that provokes allergic reactions, usually unrecognized reactions, will have a negative effect on your health.

Most vitamin pills also contain so-called inert additives that are usually not disclosed on the label. Even products thought to be the "best" contain 50 percent or more by weight of these extra ingredients. Additives are often of lower purity than the nutrients. They include lubricants, fillers, binders, and artificial colors and flavors. Unfortunately, these additives can be allergenic and toxic and can interfere with the absorption of the nutrients. For example, magnesium stearate, a lubricant, can be a potential problem. It has been proven in some cases to prevent 60 percent or more of the absorption of the nutrients in the pill, and sometimes it actually blocks absorption 100 percent. Dicalcium phosphate is another additive to avoid. It can interfere with the absorption of nutrients, even from your food. Most additives are totally unnecessary. Fillers, for example, are added to make pills bigger. Superior supplements do not contain such additives.

Supplements should be taken daily, and this is why the purity of the ingredients becomes critical. Small amounts of impurities add up over time. Every ingredient is available in a range of different purities and chemical forms. By purchasing lower-grade purity and inexpensive forms, the supplement manufacturer can save a lot of money while the consumer is none the wiser. A huge variation exists in the prices of supposedly similar vitamin products, primarily because of quality issues. The lowest acceptable purity is called "food grade," and it is the least expensive. Most popular brands are made from these low-cost, impure, food-grade ingredients. These nutrients have been found to contain toxic heavy metals, such as lead and arsenic, as well as pesticides and other harmful chemical contaminants. Consider the most common source of calcium—calcium carbonate—made from inexpensive, ground-up seashells that have been harvested from polluted waters and contain toxins. It also has very low biological activity. Only about 10 percent of the calcium is actually available for use by the body. This source of calcium is devoid of the magnesium required to help it metabolize properly, so instead of ending up in your bones, it can accumulate on your artery walls. Magnesium is often marketed as magnesium oxide, another poor choice because of low bioactivity. There are a half-dozen leading manufacturers of coenzyme (CoQ_{10}), an antioxidant and coenzyme that helps cells to produce energy. Yet only those that blend the CoQ_{10} with specific oils and other fat-soluble nutrients consistently meet high-quality standards. Meanwhile, a lot of people are taking CoQ_{10} that does not meet these standards. In 1999, a national news magazine had seven different brands of SAMe analyzed. (SAMe or S-adenosylmethionine is a molecule that all living cells produce constantly; it is involved in a fundamental biological process called methylation.) Only two products out of the seven were found to have both the correct amount and the correct chemical form of SAMe. This is what the consumer is up against.

The chemical form of a mineral that your body will use most effectively is a form that is created in combination with another compound called a transporter. The transporter enables the mineral to be transported across cell membranes and to be metabolized by your cells. Calcium citrate is an example of a good mineral form in which the citrate is the transporter. You can spot a low-quality formula when the label lists carbonates, sulfates, phosphates, and oxides because these inorganic compounds do not act as transporters, resulting in low bioactivity and depriving you of the minerals you think you are getting. Some formulas use amino acid chelates or proteinates instead of the more effective and expensive specific transporters, such as ascorbates, citrates, fumarates, and malates. While proteinates are somewhat more effective than the inorganic carbonates and oxides, they do not contain sufficient quantities of the correct transporters to be truly effective. Better formulas combine the mineral with the correct transporter in a highly purified form. Doing it right costs more, and doing it wrong gives the buyer little benefit for what they pay. See the guidelines in the next section for what to look for in a high-quality formula.

Formulated incorrectly, vitamins and minerals themselves can become toxins. Nutrients in the body are found in specific relationships. Imbalances can do more harm than good. For example, B vitamins act together in complexes that depend on these relationships. High-quality formulas respect these relationships, while poorly formulated supplements upset them, leading to an imbalance that impairs B vitamin metabolism. Most vitamin formulas contain synthetic nutrients in chemical forms that are not found in foods and are difficult for the body to excrete. That buildup can become toxic. For example, vitamin B_6 is known to be toxic in doses higher than the body needs. However, the B_6 itself is not toxic; it is the unnatural synthetic form of B_6 being used. A high-quality formula will use the correct and more expensive chemical form that is found in foods. When the correct form is used, any excess B_6 is easily removed from the body so it does not build to toxic levels. Similarly, minerals such as selenium and chromium, even at low levels, can be toxic in their inorganic forms; *their natural and more expensive organic forms eliminate the problem.* Amino acid chelates are often found in vitamin and mineral supplements, and they can contain excitotoxins that can damage the brain. *Only forms that nature uses in foods should be used in supplements,* including the transporters and cofactors that enhance the nutrient uptake from foods. Unfortunately, this rarely happens.

In the human digestive system, there are extremes of pH. In the stomach, pH is extremely acidic. Yet the absorption of nutrients takes place in the small intestine, which is an extremely alkaline environment. This range of extremes can damage nutrients and render them useless. Good-quality supplements take these considerations into account and compensate for them, but few manufacturers do this.

If a supplement contains an assortment of cheap vitamins and minerals, as these ingredients progress from the extremely acidic stomach to the extremely alkaline small intestine, they often react with each other, destroying nutrient value. Another common problem is that many supplement products mix antioxidants with oxidants in the same pill. This initiates a destructive process during the blending, production, and storage of these products, whereby valuable antioxidants such as vitamin C are destroyed by the oxidants, while the consumer has no idea this has happened. For this reason, knowledgeable manufacturers exclude oxidants such as iron, copper, iodine, sulfites, and oxidizing preservatives from their multivitamin formulas. Fortunately, this problem is easy for the consumer to check by reading the label and looking for inappropriate ingredients such as iron, copper, and iodine in their multivitamin.

Nutrients also can compete for absorption. For example, synthetic beta-carotene interferes with the absorption of other carotenes from foods. Nutrients that lose this competition pass through the body unused. To avoid these problems, the chemical forms of the nutrients must be carefully chosen to minimize competition. Again, few supplement manufacturers do this because either they lack the expertise or they are unwilling to pay for the more expensive assortment of ingredients this requires.

Consider the Source Before You Buy

To save money, some supplement manufacturers purchase old and even outdated ingredients whose potency has been diminished. How the ingredients have been shipped and stored also makes a difference. Shipping in an unrefrigerated truck in the summer and/or storage in a hot and humid warehouse damages the potency. Nutrients are also destroyed by allowing the mixed products to be exposed to oxygen, moisture, and light prior to tableting and packaging. The packaging must be done carefully and correctly to protect the nutrients until the user consumes the product.

These are just some of many considerations. When you realize how poorly most supplements are put together, it is no wonder many studies find no benefit from taking them. Raymond once advised a vitamin company he was consulting for to remove the iron from its multivitamin because the chemical form of iron they were using was reacting with and destroying the antioxidants in its formula. The company left the iron in because the marketing department thought that consumers wanted iron and that including iron on the label would be good for sales. Sadly, marketing hype and salability are paramount in the supplement industry.

Manufacturers also play games with how they list ingredients on labels. Two identical labels can contain two completely different products, one high quality, the other low quality. Without talking to the manufacturer and getting first-hand knowledge of what raw materials they are purchasing, it is not possible to know what is really in the pill. However, the following is a simple test for assessing the overall quality of a vitamin or mineral supplement. Products that do not meet this test are of low quality. Products that do meet this test may or may not be of high quality, but the probability of good quality is increased. The first thing to look at is the types of chemical compounds listed for the minerals. Look at the major minerals, such as calcium, magnesium, and zinc. What chemical form are they in? Low-quality formulas contain cheap ingredients with low absorption rates. Here is what to look for:

Low Absorption/ Bioactivity	Medium Absorption/ Bioactivity
Carbonates (e.g., calcium carbonate)	Aminoates
Oxides (e.g., magnesium oxide)	Chelates
Sulfates	Gluconates
Phosphates (except coenzyme forms)	Protein Hydrolysates

High-quality formulas contain more expensive ingredients with maximum absorption:

High Absorption/Bioactivity

Ascorbates	Malates
Citrates	Picolinates
Fumarates	Succinates
Glycinates	Tartrates

Now that you have checked the minerals, take a look at the vitamins. The easiest way to check on quality is to look at the B vitamins, specifically vitamins B_2 and B_6. In a high-quality formula, riboflavin (vitamin B_2) is accompanied by its more expensive biologically active form *riboflavin 5-phosphate*. A similar rule holds true for pyridoxine hydrochloride, vitamin B_6. A high-quality formula also contains its more expensive form *pyridoxal 5-phosphate*. These are the biologically active forms of these vitamins, and the body must convert B_2 and B_6 to these forms to be used. Since people with chronic diseases often lack the proper enzymes and have difficulty making these conversions, a good formula includes them.

Now that you are armed with knowledge about choosing high-quality supplements, let us offer a primer on why you need to supplement certain common vitamins, among them vitamins C and E. These are especially needed in order to neutralize the damaging effects of free radicals that are produced by fat cells.

Vitamin C

Vitamin C's many roles in the body are so basic to healthy function that it is almost a wonder drug. It is a powerful antioxidant, anti-inflammatory, antiviral, and anticancer compound. Vitamin C is essential to help protect against the free radicals generated by fat cells. No matter what ails you, adequate amounts of vitamin C will help. Many "incurable" conditions have been remedied simply by providing the required vitamin C.

Sadly, almost all Americans are deficient in vitamin C, which contributes significantly to our epidemic of chronic disease, including overweight. Vitamin C has the ability to donate or accept electrons easily, thereby facilitating the flow of electricity (electron flow) in the body. Electron flow controls and regulates the body's functions by promoting cell-to-cell communications. Disease happens when electron flow is impaired; life ends when electron flow stops. Insufficient vitamin C impairs flow, which is why vitamin C deficiency is a significant contributor to disease. It is also why adequate C both prevents and reverses disease. When electron flow is optimized, health and vitality are optimized. Most of us do not get enough C on a daily basis, and to make matters worse, many vitamin C supplements are potentially harmful.

According to Thomas Levy, author of *Vitamin C, Infectious Diseases, and Toxins,* "vitamin C is the single most important nutrient," and vitamin C deficiency "will facilitate the development of nearly all chronic degenerative diseases." Levy also proposes that vitamin C deficiency is the primary cause of most infectious diseases.

Infections deplete vitamin C. People who die of infections often die of complications caused by depleted vitamin C, such as internal bleeding. Levy writes, "Vitamin C is undoubtedly the ideal agent for treating any viral infection. . . . Prompt administration of very large doses of vitamin C can bring back heavily infected individuals from even comatose states, resulting in complete cures." While modern medicine administers health-damaging antibiotics and vaccinations to protect us from infections, adequate amounts of vitamin C safely prevent and eradicate almost all infectious diseases.

Vitamin C also works to neutralize the effects of toxins, which are a cause of disease. Toxins harm us by producing free radicals that damage DNA and body tissues and deplete vitamin C. Vitamin C interacts with toxins to render them harmless and also helps repair damage done by toxins. Vitamin C is the treatment of choice for virtually any toxic problem, be it snake bite, spider bite, carbon monoxide poisoning, pesticide exposure, or heavy metal poisoning.

Vitamin C may be the most important molecule we can put into our bodies to get well, stay well, and maintain optimal health. Regardless of diagnosis, vitamin C is so basic to human biochemistry that obtaining adequate amounts of vitamin C should be the foundation of any wellness strategy. Levy recommends a minimum of 6,000 mg of vitamin C per day. Most adults will need more than 6,000, perhaps 10,000 or 20,000 mg per day. Anyone with a health problem would be wise to take an amount up to what is called "bowel tolerance." To determine bowel tolerance, take vitamin C in divided doses throughout the day until excessive gas or loose stools are encountered. Reducing the dose to where this does not happen is bowel tolerance. In a healthy individual that might be 10,000 mg. In an acutely ill person, it might go as high as 100,000 mg or more.

In acute situations involving serious infections or toxic exposures, it may not be possible to obtain sufficient vitamin C orally. In these cases, intravenous vitamin C is necessary. Problems such as AIDS, cancer, carbon monoxide poisoning, hepatitis, mushroom poisoning, polio, severe acute respiratory syndrome (SARS), Lyme disease, or West Nile disease all require large doses of both oral and intravenous vitamin C. Intravenous doses of up to 50,000 to 100,000 mg per day may be necessary.

When taking large amounts of anything, make sure that what you are taking is exceptionally pure. Unfortunately, you cannot go out and just purchase vitamin C off the shelf at the health-food store. Most vitamin C is made from corn. Corn is a major allergen, and for those who are allergic to corn, corn-based vitamin C can be damaging. In addition, most vitamin

C products are not manufactured and handled with sufficient care; they often contain incorrect molecular forms, which can be irritating to the body, and oxidized vitamin C, which is a harmful free radical. Take only *corn-free, fully reduced, 100 percent L-ascorbate*—it should say this on the label.

Vitamin E

Recent years have seen an explosion of new findings on the health benefits of vitamin E. Vitamin E is particularly important to overweight individuals in order to protect against the free radicals produced by fat cells. Vitamin E appears to protect against all kinds of degenerative diseases, including cancer, heart disease, Alzheimer's disease, cataracts, and aging. Some believe vitamin E to be somewhat of a miracle drug. Dr. Evan Shute, one of the world's pioneers in vitamin E, wrote in *The Heart and Vitamin E,* "No substance known to medicine has such a variety of healing properties as E." Vitamin E has proven to be one of our most powerful biological antioxidants. The average person is deficient, but supplementing is a challenge because little "real" vitamin E is available on the market.

The two principal roles of vitamin E are as an antithrombin, to prevent blood clots inside blood vessels, and as an antioxidant, quenching free radicals linked to the development of degenerative diseases. The body employs a complex antioxidant defense system to protect itself from oxidation damage by free radicals. This system includes vitamins E, A, and C, carotenoids, bioflavonoids, gluthathione peroxidase, superoxide dismutase, alpha-lipoic acid, proanthocyanidins, and others. Unless quenched by antioxidants, free radicals can react with the fatty acids in our cell membranes, starting a chain reaction that damages the structure and function of the cell. Because vitamin E is oil-soluble, this allows it to sit right in the fatty cell membrane, protecting it from damage.

The updated RDA for vitamin E is 22 IU. Surveys indicate

that most American adults get only 12 to 15 IU. Vitamin E is found in whole grains, nuts, seeds, and fats and oils, such as authentic high-quality olive oil (most of the olive oil on the market is low-quality and adulterated). But modern diets are lacking in vitamin E because it is destroyed by cooking and processing. While even 12 IU appears to be enough to prevent obvious deficiency symptoms such as peripheral neuropathy, research indicates that many times this amount is needed for optimal health. Physicians who prescribe vitamin E usually recommend 400 IU per day for each 40 pounds of body weight, taken all at one meal. For those with critical problems, 2400 IU per day is often recommended until a regular maintenance dose is resumed.

Once deciding to supplement with vitamin E, the question becomes which brand to take. The first consideration is whether to take natural or synthetic. Synthetic E has been found to be only half as effective as natural E. There is a difference in the chemical structure of the molecules which causes synthetic vitamin E to be poorly retained by the body and less biologically active than the natural molecules. The body clearly selects the natural molecules over the synthetic, which are made from petroleum products.

When reading labels, synthetic vitamin E can usually be recognized by a "dl-" in front of the chemical name. But even products derived from natural vitamin E may not be what you want. Often natural vitamin E is reacted with organic acids to form synthetics called acetates and succinates, which are listed on the label. These acetates and succinates are stable molecules and provide long shelf life when made into supplements. The problem is these molecules are too stable and do not work well as antioxidants. In addition, they are not as well absorbed. One study found that the bioavailability of natural vitamin E was three times higher than the synthetic acetate form. There are even problems with natural vitamin E products. Most of them contain one-third to one-half vegetable oil, usually soybean, which can turn rancid and create damaging free radicals in the body.

Vitamin D

Vitamin D deficiency is one of our most common deficiencies today, and overweight people are even more prone to vitamin D deficiency than the general population. This is because fat cells absorb vitamin D and hold on to it, so it can't be used where it is needed. Up to twice as much vitamin D may be required compared to those of normal weight. If you are overweight, you need to pay special attention to your vitamin D status.

A growing body of evidence in recent years has shown that lack of vitamin D may play a vital role in heart disease, lung disease, and cancer, including colon, breast, and ovarian cancers, as well as diabetes, high blood pressure, schizophrenia, and multiple sclerosis. Vitamin D is also essential for bone health and protects against rickets in children and osteoporosis in the elderly. It has been shown to repair lung tissue and to lower insulin resistance. A review of all vitamin D studies, published in the December 2004 *American Journal of Clinical Nutrition,* found that a daily dose of vitamin D could cut the risk of cancers of the breast, colon, and ovary by up to half. The evidence for the protective effect of the "sunshine vitamin" is so overwhelming, say cancer specialists, that urgent action must be taken by public health authorities to boost blood levels.

High rates of heart disease in Scotland have been blamed on the weak sunlight and short summers in the north, leading to low levels of vitamin D. Differences in sunlight may also explain the higher rates of heart disease in England compared with southern Europe. Some experts believe the health benefits of the Mediterranean diet may have as much to do with the sun as with the regional food.

Vitamin D is made by the action of sunlight on the skin,

which accounts for 90 percent of the body's supply. But the increasing use of sunscreens and the reduced time spent outdoors, especially by children, has contributed to what many scientists believe is an increasing deficiency. Our ability to derive this vitamin from sunlight also diminishes with age.

After assessing almost every scientific paper published on the link between vitamin D and cancer since the 1960s, U.S. scientists now say that a dose of 1,000 IU (25 micrograms) is needed to maintain health. A good daily multivitamin containing vitamin D is essential. In addition, a tablespoon daily of cod-liver oil, which supplies not only vitamin D, but vitamin A and essential omega-3 fatty acids, is a good idea.

Another good idea is to periodically measure your vitamin D levels to make sure you are not deficient. Ask your doctor to measure your serum 25-hydroxyvitamin D, a simple and readily available blood test. The consensus of scientific understanding appears to be that vitamin D deficiency is reached at serum levels less than 20 nanograms per milliliter (ng/mL). Insufficiency is in the range from 20 to 32 ng/mL, and sufficiency in the range from 32 to 80. Normal in sunny countries may run between 54 and 90, and excess is greater than 100 ng/mL.

High-quality supplements play a critical role in the *NBFA* Lifestyle, helping you to achieve good health and permanent weight loss. You are now better prepared to make good selections. (For specific recommendations see Appendix D.) In the next chapter, you will learn more about how to implement this lifestyle. We provide you with six steps to help you make it part of your life.

PART IV

Implementing
the *NBFA* Lifestyle

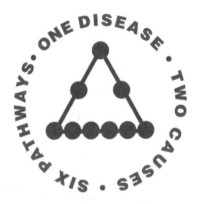

Now that you have learned the underlying causes of overweight disease, you need a plan of attack. The last two chapters are devoted to helping you take all of this new information and actually put it to work in your life at your own pace. We've divided the strategies suggested in this book into six steps, each with practical guidelines to make it easier for you. We've even provided a list for stocking your kitchen and specific meal plans to help you get started along with a wide array of delicious recipes. And don't miss the appendices, which are full of resources and helpful ideas to further assist you as you embark on a healthy, slim life.

12

STEPPING INTO
THE *NBFA* LIFESTYLE

In this chapter, you will learn more about how to implement the *NBFA* lifestyle. This chapter is packed with practical advice to get you going. Some of the topics are:

- Tips for preparing yourself and your kitchen for the lifestyle change.
- How to prepare and use your journal.
- Six steps for implementing the *NBFA* Lifestyle that you can navigate at your own pace. Each is filled with suggestions for using many of the weapons for weight loss.
- Methods for embarking on the *NBFA* Lifestyle with your family.
- Tips for eating in restaurants with the *NBFA* Lifestyle.

We have reached a point in our history where our bad

habits can no longer be tolerated. We, as a society, are on the edge of a great precipice: we can fall into sickness, poverty and degradation, or we can embrace health, longevity and bounty. All it takes is the courage to change.

—T. Colin Campbell and Thomas M. Campbell,
The China Study

Knowledge empowers change. Once your eyes are opened to new truth about what is really required to lose weight and gain health, it is difficult to live a life that denies that truth. Carrie told Michelle that when she first understood how her former diet and lifestyle affected her health she was angry because this new knowledge changed her thinking, but she was not ready to change her lifestyle. Still, she could no longer return to her former eating habits and lifestyle without a certain amount of guilt because she now knew better. Consuming toxic foods and living in careless ways lost some of its pleasure when embedded in her mind were facts that could not be denied. After trying, to no avail, to refute what she learned and enjoy her former way of living, she realized that the time had come to move forward with her newfound discoveries and adjust her lifestyle based on this truth. She shared how it then became such a joy to take responsibility for her health and build a fulfilling future. Every week people are discovering these remarkable realities, just as we once did. A new awareness dawns as we comprehend what causes over-weight along with all other manifestations of disease. This brings us to a crossroads—a time of decision.

Perhaps when you first picked up this book and began read-ing, you did not understand why you continually struggle with weight issues. You may have earnestly attempted weight loss many times and failed. Undoubtedly you believed that your weight and health concerns stemmed from "fate" or genetics, and your answers were diets, gimmicks, prescription drugs, or surgeries. After reading this life-changing, scientifically validated information, we hope the light has dawned in your mind, showing you how truly logical this approach to fighting fat as a disease is. The knowledge you have gained can empower you to step forward and transform your weight, health, and quality of life as you make lifestyle changes.

Realizing that diets fail because they are temporary and that permanent lifestyle changes can be overwhelming, we want to make the process of change manageable. These last two chapters are designed to be intensely practical to assist as you take responsibility for your weight and health. Unless you have a chronic disease that requires immediate, drastic action, you can make this lifestyle change in stages. Recall the Six Pathways that we have discussed—nutrition, toxin, mental, physical, genetic, and medical. When you begin to move steadily in the right direction on each, you cannot help but lose (pounds, of course).

We divided some of the changes on each pathway into phases or steps. Because we know many people are motivated by achieving short-term goals, we have broken these steps down into weeks. You may use this as a guide or tailor it for your situation. You choose the pace that works for you. Remember, *every step in the right direction brings you closer to better health, increased vitality, and ideal weight.* Think of it as a journey to optimal weight and health. Neither of us converted to this lifestyle overnight, nor have we "arrived." A true learner is always willing to fine-tune his or her lifestyle as science uncovers new insights about healthful living. Forging your path up a mountain can seem like a daunting challenge, but keeping your eyes focused on the next step and conquering one step at a time will enable you to reach the highest peak.

Before You Start Climbing

Before you jump in, it is a good idea to take a day or two to prepare yourself and your home for your new lifestyle. A common tendency is to prepare for a lifestyle change by wildly consuming all of the soon-to-be-forbidden foods "one last time." Perhaps the guilt is lessened when indulging with this commitment. During the holiday season, we have all heard the remark, "At the start of the New Year, I am going to make changes, so I can gorge on all of this holiday food now." The problem is that many people recite this over and over, adding countless pounds, and never getting around to *permanent* lifestyle change. This is *not* how we want you to prepare for the *NBFA* Lifestyle. Going on such a binge defeats your purpose not only by adding to the pounds that must be shed, but also by increasing toxicity and intensifying addictions. As you anticipate incorporating the *NBFA* Lifestyle, eat fewer processed foods and include more fresh, whole foods. Now is the best time to slowly decrease caffeine intake. Cut back a little more each day. If you begin to slowly reduce caffeine consumption now, it will make the transition easier when you incorporate other changes since breaking this addiction will already be under way. Rapid withdrawal from caffeine addiction is not recommended since it can result in excruciating headaches.

In preparation for the *NBFA* Lifestyle, take inventory of your mind-set, remembering what you learned in chapter 7. Concentrate on relinquishing negative thoughts and replacing them with positive expectations. Remember that the battle will be won first in your mind; therefore, you must visualize a slim and energetic you and dare to believe that you will achieve this dream. Focus on positive, bold affirmations, and choose several to use every day as you live the *NBFA* Lifestyle. Get one or two of the recommended books on the mind-body relationship from the library or bookstore. Begin to learn more about how critical it is to change your way of thinking. One new practice to include in your life is scheduling at least five minutes a day to read a minimum of a few paragraphs on nutrition and self-improvement (place a book in your bathroom if that is the only time you believe you can make). An inspiring strategy for success is to print a few motivating quotes on note cards and place them strategically around your home, and in your car and office. Make use of quotes from this book and others that will help you to stay focused and resolute.

Your Journal

Prepare your *NBFA* Lifestyle journal by enlarging the appropriate pages (see appendices B and C) and copying them on 8½-by-11 paper. You will need only one copy of Appendix B and thirty copies of the daily tracking sheets in Appendix C, one per day for each month. These can be three-hole punched and put in a monthly folder with three metal clasps, making it compact and easy to carry in a briefcase or handbag. This will be a powerful tool in assisting you to change your life.

As you envision a thin you, take a couple of full-length photographs of yourself now so you can be encouraged along the way when you compare your physical appearance to what it once was. A "before" photograph and beginning weight should be recorded on the introductory page of your journal for easy reference along with beginning measurements. We encourage you to record chest, waist, hips, and the thickest part of thigh, calf, and upper arm measurements. We would also suggest that you write down everything you eat for a couple of days before you begin. This will be interesting for you to refer back to later.

Take some time to contemplate your goals seriously and record them in your journal along with the other information on the introductory pages in Appendix B. Prepare for committed action.

Other Helps

If economics allow, now is the ideal time to request a comprehensive blood profile. A baseline test will be of great encouragement three to six months down the road when you repeat such a test and recognize the health improvement you have initiated with this lifestyle change. It will provide undeniable proof that your efforts are resulting in health benefits as well as weight loss. As we encounter clients week in and week out with health challenges, it is not uncommon to witness amazing turnarounds in cholesterol, triglycerides, blood pressure, and other blood chemistries in a relatively short period once this lifestyle is adopted.

Devise a plan for physical activity that will begin as soon as you embark on the *NBFA* Lifestyle. *We make time for what is important to us.* If you want to look and feel healthy you must make time daily for physical activity. No one will succeed without it, so exercise time must be a guarded priority. Research your options and make a plan that includes alternatives for inclement weather. Now is the time to acquire what you will need to succeed. At the very minimum, you will need some good walking shoes and a few sets of hand weights. If you have the means, a high-quality rebounder is a priority. Exercise videos, gym membership, or exercise equipment for the home are other options. Prepare for success.

Now that you have begun working on your mind by preparing your journal and planning activity, let's turn to your kitchen. Don't set yourself up for failure by embarking on your new lifestyle with a pantry and refrigerator full of your favorite processed foods. If you live with others, you may not be able to rid your home of *all* items you won't be eating, but certainly you do not want your favorite "vices" to stare you in the face when you open the refrigerator, freezer, or pantry. Get rid of them; discard them or give them away. If you are unwilling to take this step, then you are not serious about changing your life.

The day before you begin your healthy lifestyle, go shopping and stock your kitchen with fresh, organic vegetables, fruits, raw nuts, seeds, grains, and other foods you will need. Whether you use the suggested menu plans in the next chapter or devise your own, make sure you have a menu prepared. Failure occurs when you are tired at the end of the day and have no idea what to fix for dinner. This leaves you more vulnerable to the temptation to eat convenience foods. Purchase the necessary ingredients for the first few days. Gather nutritious, whole-food snacks so that they will be readily available. We recommend that you purchase some organic herbal teas, organic lemons, pure water, and stevia so that you have a constant supply of tasty drinks to accompany water between meals. Staying well hydrated with pure water will help with weight loss.

It is not a must, but consider purchases that will make your new lifestyle easier and more nutrient rich. Some helpful items include a good blender, a food processor, a high-quality juicer and/or a dehydrator (with temperature control beginning at 95 degrees to preserve enzymes). If you purchase some of these items, it may encourage you in two ways. First, you will have the capability to prepare some deliciously satisfying, enzyme-rich snacks; second, you may be more likely to continue if you have made a financial investment in your new lifestyle.

Step One (Week One): A New Beginning to the First Day of the Rest of Your Improved Life

(Note: Throughout this chapter, the asterisks in the text apply to notes following each section.)

☐ Before you set your feet upon the floor to begin the day, repeat your prepared positive affirmation(s) at least five

times with enthusiasm. Believe it. Remind yourself of
your goal: whole-body health.

☐ Make it a habit to stretch and take a couple of deep
cleansing breaths, filling your cells with oxygen as you
begin each day.

☐ Start using your journal. It may seem tedious, but it is an
incredible accountability and encouragement tool.
Record your starting weight this morning* and begin
tracking your success. Without this tool, it will be easy to
forget important practices until they become habitual.
The journal will remind you of areas where you need to
focus more attention.

☐ Start your day by drinking water. Start with a large glass
of pure water (with fresh lemon or lime and stevia, if
desired—or put in vitamin C) as soon as you rise. This
gets the system moving and helps toward your daily
water goal, often making the bowels move right away
each day. Wait at least twenty minutes after drinking this
before eating anything. It may be helpful for you to measure out your day's water in a container. This eliminates
estimating since the tendency is to believe we have had
enough when we haven't.

☐ If you are a coffee drinker, hopefully you began to cut
back in preparation for this new beginning.** Continue to
cut coffee each day and week until you are caffeine free.
Try a cup of a coffee substitute, such as Pero, Roma,
Caffix, or Teeccino (Teeccino is available in flavors and is
the only substitute that is gluten free when brewed). Don't
use decaffeinated coffee since it is toxic. Your substitute
may be mixed with smaller amounts of regular coffee
each day until you are drinking only the coffee substitute.

☐ Eliminate all sugar from your diet, along with all artificial sweeteners.***

☐ Cut back on the amount of processed food you are
consuming.****

☐ Increase your consumption of raw, living foods. Choose fresh and raw when possible. Make sure that every meal begins with raw food of some sort. We have provided a variety of salad ideas to avoid eating the same boring salad every day. If you were eating only 5 percent of your food fresh and raw, double that the first week, and aim for 10 percent the following week, and so on.

☐ Launch your fitness program.*****

Step One Notes

*Weigh yourself only one day a week and preferably at the same time of day, wearing the same amount of clothing (or no clothing). Weighing in more than once a week can be discouraging due to normal fluctuations that occur from water retention and various factors. Not weighing at all or very infrequently does not provide the encouragement and accountability needed. Knowing that you will step on the scale each Monday or each Friday acts as a motivator to keep you on track. Even if you have not had a good week, force yourself to record your weight as a reminder to get back on track. These weekly weigh-ins will encourage you as you stick to the lifestyle.

**Realize that it is not this lifestyle that is causing you to feel poorly as you break a caffeine addiction. Rather, your body has been depending upon an artificial stimulant to keep it going. You may experience some unpleasant symptoms while you are ceasing harmful addictions. You will feel better in the long run, so hang in there.

***The only sweets you should have are a couple pieces of fruit (remember that fruit is best consumed alone for breakfast or as a snack between meals, but not with other foods). When a sweetener is needed, pure stevia is the best choice. Read the labels on processed foods before you partake to be sure that they do not contain sugar in any form (use the list from chapter 2 and reread all of the information on sugar). Cold turkey is the best way to give up sugar. We don't recommend indulging in healthier sweets, other than fruit, for the first few weeks or longer.

****Replace processed foods with whole foods, beginning with snacks. Instead of reaching for processed snacks, utilize whole foods like fruit, nuts, seeds, or vegetables.

Spend more time in the produce department or at a farmers market and less time in the canned and frozen foods aisles. Replace all canned and most frozen vegetables with fresh vegetables when possible. Buy as much of your produce organic as possible. Use fresh green beans with dinner rather than canned ones and baked sweet potatoes rather than any type of processed potatoes. Get in the habit of asking, "What is the best possible choice?" Rather than choosing the boxed scalloped potatoes that are full of toxic preservatives and chemicals, buy fresh organic potatoes, and prepare a delicious dairy-free potato recipe, or just have baked potatoes. If you used to make Rice-A-Roni, replace it with a healthy brown rice pilaf recipe and significantly increase nutrition while decreasing your exposure to toxic food additives. Replace your sugar and egg-laden mayonnaise with Grapeseed Oil Veganaise, exchange sugary salad dressings for salad dressings without sugar in any form, and trade sugary ketchup for an organic health-food store brand that is unsweetened.

*****If you are not in shape physically, do not start with an intense forty-minute workout. Start with less and work your way up to a full workout. If you are in really poor shape or have never worked out, simple stretching followed by a ten-minute walk or rebounding may be all you can handle at first. If that is where you need to begin, do so, but be sure you are gradually increasing activity. Remember to utilize chapter 8 as a guideline so that you are employing all three types of exercise each week: stretching, aerobic, and weight-bearing exercise. If you have a serious amount of weight to lose, you will need to exercise three hundred minutes a week—for many, brisk walking is a good way to do this.

Step Two (Week Two): Moving On

You have made a positive start. As you implement the changes recommended in step two, continue to follow step one's changes. Stick with your journaling to provide accountability and help you to adhere to your new habits.

☐ If you followed the advice in step one and cut back on processed foods, you have already cut back on white flour. Now it is time to totally remove it. Reread the section on white flour in chapter 3 so that you will remember all of the foods containing white flour and the tips given for eliminating white flour.*

☐ Continue to reduce the processed food you are consuming. Discontinue boxed breakfast cereals and incorporate whole grains instead. Find better alternatives for all canned goods.**

☐ Step it up another notch by steadily increasing fresh, raw vegetables and fruits in your diet (organic when possible). Make it your goal to have at least half of your plate green, raw/living food at lunch and supper.***

☐ Spend time in the sunshine and fresh air every day, weather-permitting. If possible, sleep with your window open to allow your body to be nourished with fresh air while you rest. Try to exercise outdoors to accomplish three goals at once: enjoying fresh air, sunlight, and physical activity.

☐ Continue practicing all three forms of exercise: stretching, aerobics, and weight training. Strive to include scheduled exercise time at least five days a week and preferably six. If you reach a plateau with weight loss, step up the workouts to overcome it.

☐ Coach yourself with positive affirmations daily. Remember that a positive and cheerful disposition is a choice. Choose it.

☐ Continue to read material that stimulates a positive attitude and educate yourself in healthy eating and living. Remember to find time each day to read at least a few paragraphs for inspiration and motivation.

Step Two Notes

*Choose a variety of whole grains for recipes. You can use whole wheat, or even better, experiment with other whole grains such as whole oats, spelt, or kamut. Switch from regular pasta to a whole-grain variety and from processed white rice to whole-grain brown rice or another grain such as millet or quinoa.

**Eat a bowl of oats, buckwheat, or teff in place of boxed cereal. If time is an issue, use the recipe for preparing whole grains overnight in a thermos so you have a warm breakfast readily available in the morning (see chapter 13).

***Don't limit yourself to tossed salads. Experiment with some of the raw or mostly raw recipes in chapter 13 to increase raw food consumption. This is necessary for obtaining fiber and nutrients that spur weight loss and healthy cells. Expand upon raw foods by trying new recipes. Set an initial goal of half of your intake being uncooked whole foods. Eventually, 75 to 80 percent should be raw.

Step Three (Week Three): Climbing Upward!

You are halfway there in the quest to eliminate the Big Four. Continue to weigh yourself each week and journal your progress. Watch for patterns to help you discover foods that stimulate cravings, foods that don't digest well, and even circumstances that induce stress and cravings. Reread your journal to note progress and vulnerabilities.

☐ Eliminate unhealthy oils and begin including essential fatty acids. Reread the section about fats in chapter 3 as a reminder of what this step entails.*

☐ With each step you take, consume less processed food. Your grocery cart should be undergoing transformation so that it contains mostly whole foods.

☐ Along with the omission of unhealthy oils, begin every meal with uncooked food. Remember the study cited that detailed the immune response your body has to cooked foods. Eating at least half of every meal (by weight) uncooked and eating that portion first should become a habit. Think of a large salad (using a variety of salads) as the main dish.

☐ Along with healthy eating, note how many hours of sleep you are getting. Recording this in your journal each day will increase awareness of rest time. Strive for eight hours of sleep a night, especially during this time when you are losing weight and restoring health. The body heals during rest, and you can facilitate this healing.

☐ Concentrate on various ways to increase oxygen intake: living foods, aerobic workouts, breathing exercises, and sleeping in a ventilated room.**

☐ Seriously consider not just the toxins you have been putting into your body by consumption, but the toxins that you are absorbing through your skin daily. Why sabotage your progress by rubbing toxins on your permeable skin?***

☐ Remember the incredible benefits of laughter and fun. Work on becoming a fun-loving person. Laugh heartily whenever you can. Learn to enjoy life by focusing on activities rather than food.

Step Three Notes

*If you have not already done so, get rid of all vegetable oils with the exception of high-quality organic extra virgin olive oil, raw organic coconut oil, and high-quality refrigerated oils such as hemp oil and flax oil. The only ones that you should use in cooking/heating are olive oil, coconut oil, and ghee. Use flax and hemp oils strictly with uncooked recipes. Become a label reader so that you avoid toxic oils like soybean, safflower, corn, peanut, sunflower, and canola oils, which are common in processed foods. This step will help you eliminate more processed food, which is your goal.

**Living food helps to oxygenate your body, which is one reason to increase its consumption. Daily aerobic workouts must be continued since they are beneficial for increasing oxygen in your system. You can also provide more oxygen to your cells by incorporating breathing exercises in outdoor air. Take a few minutes each morning and evening to practice deep breathing. If you sleep with the window open, the evening breathing can be done as you lie in bed before falling asleep.

***Start with personal-care products. Use the guide found in Appendix D to help you find healthier options. Do not assume that a product is not toxic because it is offered at a health store; most of these products still contain toxins. One by one, switch products until you find safer alternatives for all of your personal-care needs.

Step Four (Week Four): Escalating Higher

In the next two steps, the fourth of the Big Four will be conquered. We have divided this step into two sections to make it a bit more manageable.

- ☐ Step four includes the elimination of all milk and milk products.*
- ☐ Begin to pay attention to the food combining rules you learned. As you eat foods in the proper combinations, you will maximize your energy by making the digestive

process more efficient, resulting in the assimilation of more of the nutrients consumed.**

☐ Are you still exercising daily (at least five days a week)? Your workouts should increase in intensity and duration as you become more physically fit.***

☐ In step three, you replaced toxic personal-care products; now work on better, healthier options for home-care products.****

☐ Keep your mental focus positive as you continue to climb, and avoid falling into a self-pitying frame of mind.

☐ Make sure you are keeping up with your journal and weekly weigh-ins. Take your measurements again, record them, and compare with the starting measurements.

Step Four Notes

*We recommend that you reread the sections on dairy in chapter 3 to sharpen your memory on many foods that contain dairy products. Try making the nut, seed, and grain milk recipes in chapter 13 (they are simple to prepare), and sample the banana ice cream recipe if you have not already done so. Remember that most soy, rice, and veggie cheeses still contain casein, which is a cancer-promoting milk protein. All products with casein and whey should be eliminated. This, again, will help you remove more processed foods.

**Refresh your memory on the rules of food combining:

- Eat fruit alone.
- Do not combine starchy foods with protein foods (nuts and seeds are protein).
- Vegetables can be combined with protein foods or starches.

Some people choose to make lunch a protein meal and supper a starch meal. If you follow the menu plans given in chapter 13, you will usually be adhering to proper food combinations. When you begin to launch out and plan your own menus, make sure to consider proper combinations.

***Strive to exercise for a minimum of forty-five minutes daily if health permits. Remember that the body burns fat after thirty minutes of exercise, so try to exceed that mark. Are you sweating during your workouts? Are you scheduling time for stretching, aerobic exercise, and weight training?

****Consider everything from laundry and dishwashing soaps to cleaners and air fresheners. If you have allergies and still suffer after eliminating gluten and dairy foods, you may want to purchase a recommended air purifier for your home and place it in the room where you spend the most time—most likely your bedroom.

Step Five (Week Five): Nearing the Peak

Step five is the last of the transforming steps. By taking this step, the Big Four will be completely conquered!

- ☐ It is time to let go of or greatly diminish the use of animal products other than dairy, which was eliminated in step four. This includes beef, pork, chicken, fish, and eggs along with any other meats you are consuming.*
- ☐ Continue to increase raw/living food intake steadily until your diet is 75 to 80 percent raw plant foods. At the same time, decrease processed food, which should be eaten rarely and chosen wisely when it is.
- ☐ Make sure to continue regular fitness activity. Try new routines to provide variety, which not only prevents boredom, but also awakens a variety of muscles as new exercises are undertaken. Just as a variety of healthful food is recommended, variety in exercise is also useful to ensure that all muscle groups are being worked and built.

☐ Now that you have addressed toxic personal-care products and toxic household cleaners, prescription drugs should be considered. Work with your doctor or practitioner. As your health improves your physician should assist you in eliminating most if not all of these highly toxic, health-damaging chemicals. If you have a doctor who is opposed to helping you, seek out one who will. Work toward a lifestyle that is not drug dependent. With a healthy diet and lifestyle, drugs become unnecessary, and worse, counterproductive. Natural therapies and supplements can be easily incorporated in place of almost all prescriptions.

☐ Continue to use your journal as a tool to help you live the plan. It will remind you of the various components that you should be practicing. The journal will keep you weighing in, help you to monitor your water consumption, and remind you to read, exercise, breathe deeply, stay positive, rest properly, and enjoy the sunshine. If you are not using the journal, you will not be as successful with weight loss and in maintaining all aspects of a healthy lifestyle.

Step Five Notes

*If you consume any animal products, they should be used only as condiments, not as your main course and not at every meal nor on a daily basis. Make it your practice to use vegetables and salads as the main dishes. Consider beans and lentils since they are full of fiber and nutrients. Reread the guidelines for animal products, and find an organic source for meat, poultry, eggs, and seafood. Since these sources are more expensive, this may deter you from overdosing on animal products.

Acquire a copy of *The China Study* by Dr. T. Colin Campbell from the library or bookstore. It is the most comprehensive scientific nutrition study in history, and it will motivate you to make changes. Another good motivator is a

DVD called *Eating*. Adding to your knowledge and refreshing your memory concerning what you have learned will empower you to continue this lifestyle.

If you are concerned about protein intake, remember that sprouts are loaded with amino acids and are one of the most assimilable sources of protein. Also remember that all vegetables have protein, and on a per-calorie basis, many have more than meat. One calorie worth of broccoli has almost twice the protein as one calorie of steak! Legumes, pulses, raw nuts, and seeds all provide protein.

Step Six (Week Six): Approaching the Summit at Last

Step six gives you ideas to further refine your lifestyle. If you have accomplished the previous steps, you have, no doubt, witnessed weight loss and health benefits. We hope you are convinced that this is the way you were meant to live. Feeling energetic and healthy is quite a payoff. You are nearing the summit, the highest point on the mountain, and you have made it one step at a time. But remember that you will never arrive at a point where climbing is no longer necessary.

Now that you've reached step six, consider these other *NBFA* Lifestyle options

- ☐ Add fresh vegetable and/or sprout juices and/or super-nutritious wheatgrass juice to your daily diet.*
- ☐ Fast one day a week with antioxidants from vitamin C or green juices.**
- ☐ Grow, harvest, and benefit from a variety of sprouts.***
- ☐ Dehydrate enzyme-active foods for meals and snacks.****
- ☐ Have periodic "all-raw" food days.*****
- ☐ Incorporate regular sauna times.

Step Six Notes

*"Green" juices positively affect energy level and health. Wheatgrass juice along with green juices that incorporate sprouts add significant amounts of useable protein, phytonutrients, and energizing enzymes. Many enthusiasts call wheatgrass juice the most complete food. It has only 14 calories in a two-ounce serving, but this two-ounce serving provides a gram of protein (you are hard-pressed to find any other food that provides a gram of protein in just 14 calories), and is a good source of both iron and vitamin C, not to mention the long list of benefits derived from the chlorophyll and other phytonutrients. The addition of such nutrient-dense drinks revolutionizes and supplements the diet. If you are interested, there are many books to guide you further in green juicing.

**Weekly fasting days provide many benefits, including longevity. Good books, such as *Fasting and Detoxification* by Dr. Don Colbert or *Fasting Can Save Your Life* by Herbert Shelton, will help you pursue this practice.

*** A vast variety of sprouts (broccoli, alfalfa, radish, mung bean, clover, lentil, fenugreek, adzuki, onion, cabbage, etc.) can be grown in jars and harvested year around—right in your kitchen—and they require less than five minutes a day to tend: two minutes in the morning and two minutes in the afternoon/evening to rinse them is all that is required. In four to seven days, they are ready to harvest and eat. It is simple, enjoyable, economical, and nutritious. They can be grown by those with the busiest of lifestyles and are one source of organic, raw, biogenic produce that costs only pennies per jar. When living in a cool climate, sprouts can provide you with low-cost organic produce that you know is fresh—even during the long winter.

Dr. Ann Wigmore, founder of Hippocrates Health Institute, in *The Sprouting Book* says, "The pungent cleansing sprouts, radish, fenugreek, cabbage, alfalfa, and clover are especially good for weight loss." She explains that they are not only cleansing, but are filling, nutritious, easy to digest, and low-calorie, and they speed up metabolism. They are a dieter's gold mine. Health stores sell sprouting jars with vented lids, seeds, and instructions to get you started.

****Dehydrating snacks and meals multiplies your intake of uncooked, enzyme-rich food. Well-prepared dehydrated food tastes like cooked food. Raw blended soups can be placed in the dehydrator for a short time at 105 degrees to warm them, still preserving the enzymes. Dehydrating foods can take twelve, twenty-four, or even forty-eight hours but preparation is simple and not time consuming. There are entire books on dehydrating meals and snacks, along with a few dehydrator recipes in the next chapter.

*****A great way to boost your health is to incorporate an "all-raw" food day once a week. Author and nutritionist Harvey Diamond is a firm believer in incorporating such days and even spending weeks at a time eating all raw food. Experiment with it, and find out what works for you. Remember that your body receives more nutrients and more energy from living food. Cooked food stresses the entire body.

Suggestions for scaling the heights of a healthy lifestyle are endless. Dietary pursuits certainly are not all that is involved. There are new exercise techniques, far-infrared and traditional saunas, steam rooms, whirlpools, electromagnetic therapies, massages. . . . Our list could go on and on. One never reaches the pinnacle of arriving at this healthy lifestyle. Every day there is new science from which to learn and grow. Keep expanding your knowledge.

The NBFA Lifestyle with a Family

If you are part of a family, it is likely that, especially if they have not read this book, family members will not be as eager to make changes as you may be. If you are the only one convinced that you need to change your lifestyle, use wisdom and do not forge ahead forcing changes upon unwilling spouses, parents, or children. To avoid alienating others, begin by making smaller, more subtle changes in family meals, such as switching from white bread to whole-grain bread and from white rice to brown rice. You can stop purchasing many processed foods and gradually introduce more fresh foods. Spaghetti can be made with whole-grain pasta. Once that change is accepted, switch to meatless organic sauce without unhealthy oils, added sugars, or cheese. Homemade cookies with better sweeteners and whole grains are healthier for your children than packaged, processed cookies full of white flour, sugar, bad oils, toxic additives, and dairy products. If you abruptly remove all of the "goodies," you will meet with resistance and an unhappy family. It is best not to announce a change or that what you are serving is healthier since this will cause some to automatically dislike it.

If your children are still very young, you are fortunate. Young children are usually more flexible and not as set in their unhealthy habits. We know families that raised their children this way from birth, and if it is the only way children know, they love vegetables and fresh vegetable juices and their preferred "sweet" is fruit. Teens raised this way have shared how they explored other foods in their teen years and did not like them. Their palates were not spoiled by processed foods, so they prefer healthy whole foods.

We know of a daycare center in Massachusetts where only fresh, organic, and raw vegan foods are served. Many of the families who send their children to the center are not living a healthy lifestyle. Yet most young children begin to like the food over a period of a few weeks or months. Two-, three-, and four-year-olds delightedly devour sunflower sprouts, raw vegetables, and delicious uncooked fruit pies. Often the parents notice a drastic change in the health of their children while attending this center. Chronic ear infections and frequent colds become a thing of the past. Some parents have been convinced that this must be the right way to eat by the transformed health of their little ones. This example demonstrates that, when wisely implemented, children enjoy healthier foods and benefit from them.

If you have a family, you should serve some of the food they are accustomed to along with new, healthier recipes. You can eat just the healthier options and allow them the freedom to try new things along with familiar foods. You can change without forcing the changes upon the entire family. Lead by example, but don't be pushy.

Change is more difficult with older children and teenagers. You cannot force healthy food on teenagers whom you have conditioned to eat poorly. The most you can do with older children is make organic vegetables, fruit, and other healthy options available. As you phase out processed foods, hopefully they will snack on fruit, veggies and dip, nuts, wholegrain cookies and crackers, or other healthier options. If you don't try to coerce them to change, they may try things out of curiosity or because they see you enjoying them. Your influence can have a positive affect upon them.

Restaurant Eating

More and more health-focused restaurants are popping up across the country, which is terrific for those of us who want to go out for healthy, organic fare. Most of the time you may have to eat at mainstream restaurants, but you can still make healthy choices. Limit restaurant eating to only when necessary because it will usually not be organic food and sometimes it is prepared in ways that are not health-promoting, often with added oils and toxins like MSG. Even when seeking to order the safest of food choices, it is possible that your food will still be heated in a microwave.

Almost all restaurants serve some type of salad. Look over the entire menu to access the various greens and vegetables that are used in the dishes. If you see that they have asparagus, avocado, or spinach in particular entrees, you can request these items on your salad. Ask for romaine or other leafy greens rather than iceberg lettuce. Most restaurants also serve some sort of steamed vegetables (request them without margarine or butter) and baked white or sweet potatoes. All of these are good options. Avoid eating animal products when dining out, and opt for vegetarian entrees since animal products that are not organic damage health.

Get in the habit of taking your own salad dressing with you. Most commercially prepared dressings contain sugars, processed oils, poor vinegars, and often dairy products. Don't be afraid to ask questions and mix and match from the menu. Tell the server that you are on a special diet for health challenges, and often they will go out of their way to help you. When you find a server who is willing to work with you, remember his/her name, tip well, and request that server each time.

Avoid fast-food restaurants whenever possible. If you are in a situation where you must eat fast food, look for a salad, baked potato, or the best vegetarian option possible. In any type of restaurant, avoid fried foods.

Choosing Health, Longevity, and Normal Weight

Remember, overweight is a disease—a disease that can be both prevented and reversed. Disease has only two causes: deficiency (too little of something) and toxicity (too much of something). Both deficiency and toxicity can cause our appetite and fat-storage controls to become stuck in the on position, making us constantly hungry and perpetually storing fat. Health is a choice, and you are in control.

To restore health and lose weight permanently, you must reverse deficiency and toxicity. The way to do that is to stop eating processed foods—especially the Big Four. It is not about counting calories or eating a particular diet; it is about eating real food. Switch to a natural whole-food diet consisting of fresh, organic fruits, vegetables, legumes, and unprocessed whole grains. Such a diet is automatically higher in fiber and nutrition and lower in calories and toxins. Switching to such a diet may appear difficult at first, but it is just a matter of making different choices about where and how you shop and what you buy. Add some high-quality supplements and regular exercise, and the effect on your health and weight will be almost magical.

No one in history has ever eaten the bizarre diet, been exposed to so many toxins, or lived the lifestyle that we consider to be normal. These have caused a pandemic of disease and overweight. Reversing this pandemic requires a long-term commitment. Any effort that does not include permanent lifestyle changes will fail. At this very moment, you are determining your future health and weight destiny. It is not preordained for you to be overweight, to watch your health decline as you grow older, or to live a lifetime of compromised health. Each of us has the choice of doing nothing or doing something. Too many of us end up doing the wrong thing or nothing because we don't know what to do. Few of us have ever been taught how to choose health over disease, which is why most of us are sick and overweight. We have been making uninformed choices, unwittingly choosing overweight, disease, and premature death. There is even a new medical term to describe these poor choices and the diseases they create— "lifestyle syndrome." We can stop doing it wrong right now and start planning our own health destiny. It is the most important and loving thing you can do for yourself.

To adopt a new way of living, use the Six Pathways to move yourself toward optimal health and weight on the health and disease continuum. The body knows how to keep us healthy and control our weight. Our job is to help it to do so. Achieving optimal health and weight doesn't mean you have to do everything perfectly. What you eat in a week is more important than what you eat at one meal. The cumulative effect of doing it right most of the time can be as beneficial as having done it wrong most of the time has been harmful. What is essential is establishing and maintaining healthy lifestyle habits that you enjoy and want to be part of your life and the way you live.

You cannot accomplish your goals without making a commitment. Even if you focus on one pathway per week or month, in six weeks or at most six months you will have your new lifestyle in place. Take responsibility for your life— choose the *NBFA* Lifestyle. If you do this, you will achieve a substantial and healthy reduction in weight while helping to prevent and reverse a host of chronic diseases. Don't wait until you are facing a life-threatening disease to take action.

As you continue to learn, you will continue to make new healthy changes. We would love to hear from you and be made aware of your successes with the *NBFA* Lifestyle (contact information appears in Appendix A).

Never be fat again. Stop dieting, and lose weight!

13

NBFA MENUS, RECIPES, AND KITCHEN HELPS

This chapter is designed to help you to survive and even enjoy the *NBFA* Lifestyle. These meal plans and recipes provide you with options to replace the destructive fare we have suggested that you eliminate. It would be cruel for us to tell you that what you are eating is making you fat and sick and then not teach you how to change. This practical chapter shows you how to fight fat as a disease and change your life for the better. Among the information you'll read in this chapter:

- Raw vegetables are much more than just tossed salads. You'll discover many meals based upon raw vegetable delights.
- Main dishes can be made without meat, poultry, or fish—learn how.

- Doing without milk and cheese is one of the hardest alterations for most people—we will show you how.

Food is meant to be enjoyed every day as a celebration. No one has to give up the pleasure of eating in order to become healthy.

—Frederic Patenaude
Sunfood Cuisine

This chapter offers sample menu plans, including delicious recipes that take you back to the basics—fresh, whole food—to get you started with the *NBFA* Lifestyle. Since you now understand what makes a healthy diet, you can transform your own recipes. You can remake old favorites by replacing processed ingredients and the Big Four with better alternatives. Some of your revised recipes will be better than the originals.

When making substitutions, lentils can easily replace ground beef in recipes. Often organic portobello mushrooms can replace steak or chicken, such as in the "Where's the Beef?" Bul Go Gee. Chicken and beef broths may be replaced with vegetable broths. Always try to replace canned products with their fresh counterparts. If this is impossible, use frozen.

Sometimes simple is best. If you stick to whole foods in their unprocessed form, you have real fast food. You don't have to cook up a storm to have a meal. Some fruit and a handful of nuts can be breakfast on a busy morning. A simple sweet potato, baked or steamed along with a salad is an easy supper on a hectic evening. As you transition, you may want more elaborate recipes at the beginning, which is normal. But it is freeing to know that you can always fall back on simple, nutritious whole foods.

Menu Plans

We have included three sets of sample menus. One is for those who are transitioning from a Standard American Diet. This set of meal plans incorporates whole foods as the basis of the diet, with about half of the intake as raw vegetables, fruits, nuts, and seeds. The second set of menus represents a diet with a higher percentage of raw food. The third is a menu plan for one all-raw day, since people often ask us how a person can eat all raw food.

Obviously a new lifestyle will take some learning. Be patient and allow time for adjustment to preparing and enjoying new types of food. Don't give up just because some effort is required on your part to go from a diet of mostly processed food to a diet of whole foods. You will lose some convenience as you gain health and lose weight. Clearly, giving up canned goods and ready-to-eat foods and using whole foods will mean a totally different way of meal preparation. Driving through fast-food restaurants will be replaced by Crock-Pot dinners that can be ready when you arrive home, but they require advance planning and a few minutes of extra preparation time. Remembering what is at stake—your health—will make the changes worth the effort. Planning is the name of the game when applying what you have learned on the Nutrition Pathway. The foods are not difficult to make, but it is critical that you plan ahead, drafting menus for at least a few days at a time. This preparation ensures that you have the necessary ingredients on hand, soaked (if necessary), and ready to use in the recipes. The menus are arranged so that you can utilize leftovers and prepare basics that can be used for several meals. For example, once you make the burritos with meatless taco "meat," the leftover taco "meat" can be used for a taco salad the following day for lunch.

Another example is soaking and boiling a large batch of garbanzo beans so that you can prepare hummus (which can be refrigerated for about five days) and have enough garbanzos left for a garbanzo bean salad, and the remainder can be used as a salad topping.

Sample Daily Menus

You may always substitute another fruit for any fruit not in season or not available.

An asterisk (*) denotes that the recipe follows the menu plans. Recipes are listed in the order in which they appear in the menu plans.

The evening before beginning: Prepare the thermos grain for the morning.

For day one, purchase organic hummus with no added oils, or make a batch of your own (see page 295).

Your Rising Routine Beverage (to be used every day)

Upon rising, drink a large glass or two of fresh water. This can be plain water, water with vitamin C, or lemon water, with or without stevia (lemon is good for the liver).

Phase One Menu (Transition Diet)/Day One

Rising Routine Beverage

Soak one cup of organic lentils in two cups of pure water for the day to reduce cooking time for the meatless taco "meat" tonight.

Breakfast (If you prepare this in a thermos, you can take it with you to work if you are not hungry first thing in the morning.)
No-Cook Breakfast Delight (see page 292) with 1 tablespoon ground flaxseed and milk alternative (see page 293) if desired; may be topped with stevia, cinnamon, and nutmeg

Snack   A ripe apple or peach, or cup of blueberries with or without a handful of raw nuts

Lunch   Build Your Own Veggie Sandwich (see page 294)
            An acceptable (no added oils, MSG, etc.) whole-
            grain cracker and hummus (see page 295)
Snack   Large serving of watermelon or raw assorted veggies
Dinner Basic Tossed Green Salad with Creamy South-
            western Dressing (see page 297)
            NBFA Burritos with Meatless Taco "Meat" (see page 298)
            (Try to make the salad large and focus on it, eating
            only one burrito afterward.)

Phase One Menu (Transition Diet)/Day Two

Rising Routine Beverage

Breakfast Bowl of No-Cook Breakfast Delight (see page
            292) with milk alternative, if desired
Snack   Leftover hummus with baby carrots and healthier
            crackers to dip
Lunch   *NBFA* Taco Salad (see page 298) with leftover taco
            "meat"
Snack   ½ honeydew melon or cantaloupe
Dinner Caesar Salad (see page 302)
            Veggie Pasta (see page 303)

Phase One Menu (Transition Diet)/Day Three

Rising Routine Beverage

Marinate the portobellos for tonight's "Where's the Beef?"
Bul Go Gee (see page 308)
Soak 2 cups of brown rice in 4 cups of water for tonight's meal
to reduce preparation time.

288 Implementing the *NBFA* Lifestyle

Breakfast	Ezekiel Sprouted Grain Bagel or toasted Manna Bread with coconut oil or Healthier Spread* (see page 304)
Snack	Apple slices with a handful of almonds or raw, organic almond butter
Lunch	Raw veggies with Vegan Ranch Dressing as dip (see page 305)
	Build Your Own Veggie Sandwich (see page 294)
Snack	Creamy Banana Milk Shake (see page 306) smoothie, or a cup of cherries
Dinner	Colorful Cabbage Delight* (see page 306)
	"Where's the Beef?" Bul Go Gee* (see page 308) served over brown rice

On a day when you have extra time, be adventurous and experiment with vegetable juice in the morning, before eating. Kick start your day by putting any mixture of vegetables through the juicer. Initially you may add two organic apples to help you tolerate the taste. Slowly reduce to one apple. It tastes like apple juice, yet you get an incredible antioxidant boost along with numerous minerals, vitamins, and phytochemicals.

Sample Daily Phase Two Menus (Larger Percentage Raw Food)

Please keep in mind that the salads served at meals in this plan are large and should be the prominent part of the meal. The other dish is eaten as a side item. This is opposite of the way most of us are accustomed to eating—with a side salad and a plateful of cooked food. One good practice is to use a large plate for the fresh salad and a salad plate or bowl for the other part of the meal. This will train you to reverse your typical eating pattern.

Phase Two
Menu (Larger Percentage Raw Food)/
Day One

Rising Routine Beverage

Breakfast A bunch of grapes and ¼ cup raw sunflower seeds

Snack   Sliced veggies with Guacamole (see page 299)

Lunch   Large Basic Tossed Green Salad (see page 296)
             with dressing of choice
             Mexican Sandwich Filling (see page 309) wrap or
             sandwich

Snack   Celery with raw almond butter and ground
             flaxseed sprinkled on top

Dinner   Romaine with Lemon Dulse Dressing (see page 310)
             Steamed green beans or asparagus

Phase Two
Menu (Larger Percentage Raw Food)/
Day Two

Rising Routine Beverage

Soak beans for Day Three Cincinnati Chili recipe

Breakfast Cinnamon Buckwheat Cereal* (see page 312) with
              milk alternative

Snack   Two kiwis and a handful of raw pistachios

Lunch   Versatile Veggie Wraps (see page 312) or leftover
             Mexican Sandwich Filling with whole-grain
             tortillas or wrapped in a romaine or collard leaf
             instead of bread
             Assorted raw vegetables or tossed salad

Snack   Healthy Lifestyle Ice Cream (see page 314)

Dinner   Large Tossed Salad with Italian Olive Oil Dressing
                (see page 314)
                Veggie Pesto Pasta (see page 315)

If you are away during the daytime, while cleaning up after
dinner, start the Meatless Cincinnati Chili with pasta* (see
page x) for tomorrow's dinner. It can be refrigerated and put
in the Crock-Pot on low all day tomorrow to finish cooking.

Phase Two
Menu (Larger Percentage Raw Food)/
Day Three

Rising Routine Beverage

Put the Cincinnati Chili ingredients (except the pasta and extra
onions) in the Crock-Pot on low before leaving for the day.

Breakfast Favorite Tropical Smoothie (see page 319) and a
                Banana Nut and Seed Bar (see page 320)
Snack   Spicy Raw Nuts (see page 321)
Lunch   Tossed salad with dressing of choice
                Ripe organic avocado half
                Healthy whole-grain cracker without oil
Snack   Assorted vegetables with hummus or salad dress-
                ing of choice
Dinner   Yellow Squash Carrot Salad (see page 322)
                served on a bed of greens and/or sprouts
                Meatless Cincinnati Chili (see page 317) with
                whole-grain pasta (freeze the leftover chili for use
                as a quick meal on a busy evening)

Sample Daily Phase Three Menu (All-Raw)

After you get acclimated to the *NBFA* Lifestyle, you may desire to try "living food days" once a week and eat all of your food uncooked. This gives your body a boost of energy and nutrients. Here is a sample of how you might choose to eat on such a day. Remember, the goal is to eat 75 to 80 percent of your food raw.

Phase Three (All-Raw)

Rising Routine Beverage

Breakfast Uncooked Whole-Grain Buckwheat Breakfast
(see page 323) with cinnamon, nutmeg, and stevia
1 tablespoon ground flaxseed
Milk alternative (see page 293)

Snack Veggie Flax Crackers (see page 323) with
Guacamole (see page 299)

Lunch Mexican Cabbage Salad (see page 324)
Veggie Flax Crackers

Snack Two plums and a handful of raw almonds

Dinner Large tossed salad
Tantalizing Trio Salad (see page 326)
Brazil Nut Loaf (see page 328) or if you don't
have a dehydrator, eat it unheated as paté served
on a bed of greens or a romaine leaf

R E C I P E S

Phase One/Day One

No-Cook Breakfast Delight (phase 1)

Place wheat berries, buckwheat, quinoa, or oats in a thermos the evening before you plan on eating them. Boil pure water and place the correct amount of boiling water in the thermos with the grain. (See chart on next page for correct amounts of grain and water.) If you wish, you may combine some cinnamon, nutmeg, and stevia with the grain at this point, or it can be added in the morning. Promptly put the lid on the thermos and let sit until morning when the grain will be ready to eat without cooking. Stir and enjoy.

An ideal way to introduce ground flaxseed into your diet is by sprinkling it on top of a bowl of whole grains. Using a coffee grinder, grind 1 tablespoon of flaxseed to top your whole grains.

Cereal and Grain Preparation

Rather than using boxed cereals, which are highly processed and have little nutrition, try incorporating various whole grains for breakfast. All grains may be seasoned with cinnamon and stevia and served with a milk substitute. If time is a concern for cooking grains, try an overnight method and your grains will be ready to eat when you get up in the morning.

If you plan ahead and soak grains in pure water prior to usage, this makes them much easier to digest. Cooking time is reduced since this soaking softens the grains. Some grains, such as buckwheat, can be soaked overnight and then eaten without cooking. They are soft and ready to eat after soaking or may be cooked if you desire.

Here is a general guide for grain cooking. Bear in mind that soaked grains may cook in less time and may require slightly less water.

Grain	Dry Amount	Water	Cooking Time
Brown rice	½ cup	1 cup	45–50 minutes
Buckwheat	½ cup	1 cup	30–35 minutes
Millet	½ cup	1½ cups	40 minutes
Oats (groats)	1 cup	2½ cups	40–60 minutes
Quinoa	½ cup	1 cup	20 minutes
Teff	½ cup	2 cups	20 minutes
Wheat	½ cup	1 cup	60 minutes

Regular Stove-Top Cooking

Bring the water to a boil. Add grain, cover, reduce heat, and simmer until soft. It is best not to remove the lid or stir whole grains during the cooking time.

Almond, Walnut, Sesame Seed, Sunflower Seed, Pumpkin Seed, or Buckwheat Milk

> ½ cup nuts, seeds, or buckwheat
> 2 cups pure water
> a pinch of pure stevia exract powder
> ¼ teaspoon alcohol-free vanilla (optional)

Soak the nuts, seeds, or buckwheat of your choice overnight. Drain.

Place in blender and grind until fine. Add half of the water and the sweetener, and blend again until it is creamy (less than a minute). Slowly pour the remaining water through the hole in the blender lid while the blender is still running on high. Blend until mixed.

Pour the mixture into a cheesecloth or very fine strainer over a bowl or glass measuring cup (a nut milk bag is the easiest to use for this and can be acquired from www.hippocratesinst.org; click on "Store"). Allow the milk to filter through the strainer. Squeeze the cloth or bag after all of the milk has passed through, wringing it out.

The milk will keep in the refrigerator for four or five days. The pulp may be used in other recipes, such as nut loaf, veggie burgers, and muffins, or dried for use as a sprinkle for salads. (Dehydrated almond pulp is used in the Caesar Salad recipe.)

This recipe may be doubled for larger amounts of milk.

(Add ¼ teaspoon vanilla if you want to make vanilla milk—this is good when preparing something sweet or pouring the milk on cereal or cooked grain.)

MAKES APPROXIMATELY 2 CUPS (SERVING SIZE ½ CUP)

Calories: 80 • Calories from fat: 60 • Total fat: 7g
Saturated fat: 0.5g • Trans fat: 0g • Cholesterol: 0mg
Sodium: 0mg • Total Carbohydrate: 3g
Dietary Fiber: 2g • Sugars: 1g • Protein: 3g
Nutritional content may vary depending upon preparation.

Build Your Own Veggie Sandwich

Vegenaise or organic mustard (or both, depending upon your
    preference)
2 slices whole-grain bread (preferably sprouted) or sprouted-grain wrap
vegetables of your choice: sliced tomato, avocado, cucumber
greens of your choice: romaine, leaf lettuce, spinach
sprouts, any varieties
sea salt to taste

Spread the Veganaise or mustard on bread or lightly toasted bread. Top with vegetables and greens of choice. Top with sprouts and sprinkle with sea salt. Enjoy a healthier alternative to a meat and cheese sandwich.

MAKES 1 SERVING

Calories: 280 • Calories from fat: 70 • Total fat: 8g*
Saturated fat: 0g • Trans fat: 0g • Cholesterol: 0mg
Sodium: 450mg • Total Carbohydrate: 45g
Dietary Fiber: 7g • Sugars: 5g • Protein: 9g
*4 grams fat from spelt bread and 4 grams from Vegan mayo
Nutritional content may vary depending upon preparation.

Garlicky Herbed Hummus

Many packaged hummus blends contain unhealthy oils and are not recommended. One acceptable brand is Nature's Healthy Gourmet, which has no added oil. If you have a food processor, it is easy to make your own hummus.

1½ cups organic garbanzo beans
1 tablespoon raw organic sesame tahini
juice of one organic lemon (approximately ½ cup)
2 cloves fresh garlic, minced
½ teaspoon sea salt
½ cup Beyond Health Olive Oil (I omit the oil many times)
Reserved cooking water to desired consistency (about ¼–½ cup)
fresh herbs of any combination you enjoy—options include basil,
    parsley, oregano, dill, and cilantro
Either red pepper or tomato can be added for variety

Soak the beans in pure water overnight or all day, then drain. Cook the beans in fresh pure water until tender (40–60 minutes). Drain the beans, reserving the cooking water, and cool slightly. Combine the beans, tahini, lemon juice, garlic, sea salt, and just enough of the reserved water in a food processor until smooth. Pour the olive oil through the chute while processing. Pulse the herbs, tomato, or red pepper into the mixture if you are using them.

Store your hummus in the refrigerator, preferably in a glass container. It will keep for up to five days.

Use the hummus as a vegetable dip, eat it on crackers (raw or whole-grain packaged), or put it on wraps.

MAKES ABOUT 2 CUPS

Calories: 100 • Calories from fat: 70 • Total fat: 8g*
Saturated fat: 1g • Trans fat: 0g • Cholesterol: 0mg
Sodium: 75mg • Total Carbohydrate: 5g
Dietary Fiber: 1g • Sugars: 1g • Protein: 2g
Nutritional content may vary depending upon preparation.

Basic Tossed Green Salad

Begin with a mixture of organic greens. Try to include at least three or four different greens for variety. Some of our favorites are

Boston lettuce
green leaf lettuce
kale (not the curly variety, but the newer flat, Lacinto variety)
red leaf lettuce
romaine (We prefer the entire romaine "head" and not just the
     hearts. The outer leaves contain the most chlorophyll. When
     you purchase just the hearts, you miss those quality leaves.)
spinach
Swiss chard
watercress

Wash the greens, tear them up, and place them in a salad spinner (a good salad spinner is well worth the investment when salad is something you eat daily).

Choose as many of the following organic salad toppings as you like and have on hand:

artichokes	garbanzo beans	shredded carrots or
asparagus	jicama	sweet potato
avocado	mushrooms	shredded raw beets
broccoli florets	pumpkin or sun-	slivered almonds
cauliflower	flower seeds	snow peas or sugar
celery	radishes	snap peas
cucumber	red cabbage, sliced	tomato
fresh sprouts of all	red or white onion	zucchini or yellow
varieties	red or yellow pepper	squash

Toss toppings with greens and serve.

With such variety, there is no reason for your salads to be the same every day.

Calories: 70 • Calories from fat: 35 • Total fat: 4g*
Saturated fat: 0g • Trans fat: 0g • Cholesterol: 0mg
Sodium: 10mg • Total Carbohydrate: 7g
Dietary Fiber: 3g • Sugars: 4g • Protein: 3g
Includes 1 tbsp of nuts and seeds
Nutritional content may vary depending upon preparation.

Creamy Southwestern Dressing

1 cup salsa (if it is store bought, make sure you find an organic
   option without sugar or MSG in any of its forms)
2 tablespoons Vegenaise Grapeseed Oil Dressing (available in
   health-food stores)

Mix the above and add some fresh herbs, such as oregano, cilantro, basil, parsley, or dill if desired.

MAKES 8 SERVINGS

Calories: 10 • Calories from fat: 5 • Total fat: 0.5g
Saturated fat: 0g • Trans fat: 0g • Cholesterol: 0mg
Sodium: 160mg • Total Carbohydrate: 1g
Dietary Fiber: 0g • Sugars: 0g • Protein: 0g
Nutritional content may vary depending upon preparation.

Meatless Taco or Burrito "Meat"

This recipe can be used to replace the ground beef commonly used on taco salads or in burritos. You can make a large batch and serve it in burritos, then use the leftovers cold for taco salad the following day. It is delicious, and some people do not even realize that it is not ground beef!

1 large onion, chopped
2 cloves of garlic, pressed into the skillet
1 tablespoon Beyond Health Olive Oil
1 cup dry organic lentils, soaked for several hours or overnight
    (You can skip the soaking if you have not planned ahead, but it
    is far better to soak.)
1 tablespoon chili powder
1 tablespoon ground cumin
1 teaspoon dried oregano
¼–½ teaspoon sea salt (depending on taste)
2 cups pure water (½ cup less if lentils have been soaked)
½ cup organic salsa (homemade or carefully selected)

In a large skillet, sauté the onion and garlic in olive oil until tender. While they are sautéing, drain and rinse the lentils. Add the lentils, along with all of the spices, to the skillet and sauté, stirring for another couple of minutes. Add the water and bring it back to a boil. Reduce heat, cover, and simmer until the water has diminished and lentils are tender, about 30 minutes. Remove the lid and continue cooking until the rest of the water is evaporated and the mixture is thickened. Mash the lentils slightly with a potato masher. You do not want them totally mashed, but rather a chunky consistency. Add the salsa and mix thoroughly. Serve and use as you would use taco meat.

MAKES 6–8 WRAPS; 4 TACO SALAD SERVINGS

Calories: 240 • Calories from fat: 45 • Total fat: 5g*
Saturated fat: 0.5g • Trans fat: 0g • Cholesterol: 0mg
Sodium: 320mg • Total Carbohydrate: 36g
Dietary Fiber: 7g • Sugars: 3g • Protein: 13g
Nutritional content may vary depending upon preparation.

NBFA Burritos

6–8 Sprouted Ezekiel Tortillas or Food for Life Brown Rice
   Tortillas
1 recipe Meatless Taco "Meat" (see preceding recipe)
freshly chopped onion
freshly chopped tomatoes
shredded romaine or other lettuce
sliced avocado (or Guacamole; see next recipe)
salsa (organic and without sugar or MSG)

Lay the tortilla on a plate. Place ⅓ cup of the lentil mixture across
the center, going all the way to one edge and leaving 1 inch at the
opposite edge. Place desired toppings on the lentils. Fold the end
where you left the one-inch margin over first, then fold the two sides
inward, forming a burrito. Warning: if you overfill it, it will be difficult to handle.

MAKES 6–8 SERVINGS

Calories: 450 • Calories from fat: 90 • Total fat: 10g*
Saturated fat: 0.5g • Trans fat: 0g • Cholesterol: 0mg
Sodium: 580mg • Total Carbohydrate: 69g
Dietary Fiber: 10g • Sugars: 4g • Protein: 19g
Based on Sprouted Ezekiel Tortillas
Nutritional content may vary depending upon preparation.

Guacamole

2 ripe avocados, peeled and mashed
¼ cup finely diced onion
1 large clove garlic, minced
2 tablespoons fresh-squeezed lime juice
1 small tomato, chopped well
dash of cayenne powder
sea salt to taste

In a glass bowl, mash all of the ingredients together, leaving it
chunky if you desire. For a smoother combination, you can put it all
in the food processor and blend.

Serve in your favorite Mexican recipe, on vegetables, or on crackers.

Tip: A ripe avocado is dark in color and not mushy, but gives to pressure. If you get avocados that are not ready to use, leave them out at room temperature until they ripen. To cut an avocado, use your knife to cut all the way around the seed, cutting it in half long ways. Placing one hand on each half, twist to open the avocado. To remove the pit, put the knife into the pit and twist. If your avocado is ripe the pit will come out. If you do not use the entire avocado, it will turn brown. Leaving the pit in the unused portion and wrapping it helps to preserve it for a longer period of time.

MAKES 6–8 SIDE SERVINGS

Calories: 110 • Calories from fat: 90 • Total fat: 10g
Saturated fat: 1.5g • Trans fat: 0g • Cholesterol: 0mg
Sodium: 5mg • Total Carbohydrate: 8g
Dietary Fiber: 5g • Sugars: 1g • Protein: 2g
Nutritional content may vary depending upon preparation.

Phase One/Day Two

NBFA Taco Salad

3-4 cups mixed salad greens
1 large organic onion, chopped
1 large organic cucumber, chopped
1 large organic red pepper, chopped or sliced
1–2 ripe avocados, peeled and chopped
1 cup organic grape tomatoes (unless the tomatoes in the salsa are
    enough for you)
fresh homemade salsa or healthy organic salsa
1 recipe Meatless Taco "Meat" (see recipe page 298)

Clean salad greens and distribute them among four plates.

Top each plate of greens with onion, cucumber, red pepper, and tomatoes.

Make a "well" in the center of each plate. Scoop ¾ cup of the Meatless Taco "Meat" into each well. Cover salad with a liberal amount of homemade salsa. Distribute chopped ripe avocado over salad. Enjoy!

MAKES 4 SERVINGS

Calories: 380 • Calories from fat: 120 • Total fat: 13g
Saturated fat: 2g • Trans fat: 0g • Cholesterol: 0mg
Sodium: 470mg • Total Carbohydrate: 53g
Dietary Fiber: 14g • Sugars: 9g • Protein: 16g
Nutritional content may vary depending upon preparation.

Caesar Salad

Adapted from Ken Blue's recipe. Ken is executive chef at Hippocrates Health Institute.

1 head romaine lettuce, torn in bite-sized pieces
¼ red onion, diced
1 carrot, shredded
1 cup almond meal* (or ground almonds)
½ cup dried hijiki** soaked in water and drained (optional)

Mix all of the above in a large glass bowl and toss with dressing.

MAKES 4 LARGE SERVINGS

Calories: 190 • Calories from fat: 110 • Total fat: 12g
Saturated fat: 1g • Trans fat: 0g • Cholesterol: 0mg
Sodium: 35mg • Total Carbohydrate: 15g
Dietary Fiber: 6g • Sugars: 6g • Protein: 8g
Nutritional content may vary depending upon preparation.

Caesar Salad Dressing

1 clove garlic, minced
⅛ cup extra virgin olive oil
1 tablespoon fresh lemon juice
½ cup raw sesame tahini
½ teaspoon mustard powder
2 tablespoons kelp powder***
1 tablespoon fresh oregano, minced
½–⅔ cup pure water

In a blender, combine all of the dressing ingredients except the water. Blend until very smooth. Add water to adjust consistency.

Toss this dressing with the salad and enjoy.

*Almond meal is what is left behind after preparing almond milk. Instead of throwing this pulp in the garbage or compost, put it in your dehydrator at 105°F (or in a very low oven) and leave it until it becomes crunchy. Store it in the refrigerator. It makes a delicious salad additive. If you do not have almond meal use ground almonds.

**Hijiki is a sea vegetable. It is full of minerals and tasty, but does not have to be added. You can try using just a little at a time until you acquire a taste for sea vegetables.

***Kelp powder is finely ground kelp (a sea vegetable) that can be purchased at a health store and adds saltiness and flavor.

MAKES 4 SERVINGS

Calories: 270 • Calories from fat: 220 • Total fat: 25g
Saturated fat: 3.5g • Trans fat: 0g • Cholesterol: 0mg
Sodium: 10mg • Total Carbohydrate: 9g
Dietary Fiber: 5g • Sugars: 0g • Protein: 7g
Nutritional content may vary depending upon preparation.

Veggie Pasta

3 cloves garlic, minced
1 bunch green onions, chopped
2 tablespoons fresh basil, chopped
2 tablespoons fresh oregano, chopped
2 tablespoons fresh parsley, chopped
⅓ cup Beyond Health Olive Oil
1 package Tinkyada brown rice pasta (or whole-grain spaghetti or pasta of choice)
2 cups fresh organic broccoli, chopped
1 large onion, sliced in rings
1 cup organic baby carrots, julienned
1½ cups chopped organic asparagus
1 small zucchini, chopped
1 small yellow squash, chopped
1 cup chopped organic shitake mushrooms (optional)
2 large ripe organic tomatoes, chopped
sea salt to taste
¼ cup Soymage Parmesan Cheese (optional, available at health-food stores)

Place the garlic and fresh herbs in the olive oil in a glass bowl and let it soak while you chop and prepare the other ingredients.

Boil the pasta. While the pasta is boiling, prepare a large Dutch oven for steaming, and steam the chopped broccoli, onion, carrots, asparagus, zucchini, yellow squash, and mushrooms.

When the pasta is cooked, drain. Toss the steamed veggies with the hot pasta. Add the fresh uncooked tomatoes, and the olive oil mixed with herbs and garlic. Toss it all together, salt to taste, and serve immediately. If desired, add Soymage sprinkle.

MAKES 6–8 SERVINGS

Calories: 250 • Calories from fat: 100 • Total fat: 11g
Saturated fat: 2g • Trans fat: 0g • Cholesterol: 0mg
Sodium: 65mg • Total Carbohydrate: 32g
Dietary Fiber: 4g • Sugars: 4g • Protein: 6g
Nutritional content may vary depending upon preparation.

Phase One/Day Three

Healthier Spread

¼ cup Beyond Health Olive Oil
¼ cup organic, raw, virgin coconut oil
½–1 teaspoon sea salt (depending upon taste)

In a small glass jar, combine all ingredients. Close the jar and shake well. Refrigerate and use in place of butter as a spread. You may use less coconut oil and more olive oil if you prefer the taste.

MAKES ABOUT 20 SERVINGS

Calories: 45 • Calories from fat: 45 • Total fat: 5g
Saturated fat: 2.5g • Trans fat: 0g • Cholesterol: 0mg
Sodium: 50mg • Total Carbohydrate: 0g
Dietary Fiber: 0g • Sugars: 0g • Protein: 0g
Nutritional content may vary depending upon preparation.

Vegan Ranch Dressing

Mix the following in a 2-cup glass measuring cup:

1½ cups Vegenaise Grapeseed Oil Dressing
2 teaspoons organic apple cider vinegar
2 cloves fresh garlic, minced
½ teaspoon garlic powder
½ teaspoon onion powder
fresh herbs of your choosing: try parsley, oregano,
  basil, dill, or marjoram

Mix all of the above in a 2-cup glass measuring cup. Add herbs liberally. If you do not have fresh herbs, you may use dried ones. Thin mixture with nut milk, rice milk, or a little bit of pure water to desired consistency. A little liquid goes a long way in thinning this dressing, so stir in your liquid a little at a time. For vegetable dip, leave the mixture thicker.

Optional: To make a cheesy ranch, you may add 1 tablespoon Soymage Vegan Parmesan or 1 tablespoon nutritional yeast.

MAKES 1¾ CUPS

Calories: 15 • Calories from fat: 15 • Total fat: 1.5g
Saturated fat: 0g • Trans fat: 0g • Cholesterol: 0mg
Sodium: 45mg • Total Carbohydrate: 0g
Dietary Fiber: 0g • Sugars: 0g • Protein: 0g
Nutritional content may vary depending upon preparation.

Creamy Banana Milk Shake

2 frozen bananas (freeze for at least 24 hours)
1 cup almond milk or other milk substitute
⅛ teaspoon vanilla

Blend until smooth and serve. So creamy and delicious, you won't miss the milk.

You can make this into a carob milk shake by adding a tablespoon of unsweetened carob powder and a small amount of pure stevia extract powder to taste.

You can adapt this recipe by adding other fruits along with the banana, but keep at least 1½ bananas as the base for creaminess.

MAKES 2 SERVINGS

Calories: 240 • Calories from fat: 35 • Total fat: 3.5g
Saturated fat: 0g • Trans fat: 1g • Cholesterol: 0mg
Sodium: 160mg • Total Carbohydrate: 54g
Dietary Fiber: 6g • Sugars: 32g • Protein: 3g
Nutritional content may vary depending upon preparation.

Colorful Cabbage Delight

2 cups shredded or grated cabbage (may be partly red cabbage, if
    desired)
½ cup shredded jicama
½ cup shredded carrot
½ cup chopped red bell pepper
¼ cup diced onion (red onion is eye appealing)
¼ cup diced celery

Toss all of the above vegetables in a bowl.

MAKES 2 LARGE SERVINGS

Calories: 60 • Calories from fat: 0 • Total fat: 0g
Saturated fat: 0g • Trans fat: 0g • Cholesterol: 0mg
Sodium: 45mg • Total Carbohydrate: 14g
Dietary Fiber: 5g • Sugars: 6g • Protein: 2g
Nutritional content may vary depending upon preparation.

Dressing

½ cup raw apple cider vinegar
1 clove garlic, minced
⅛ teaspoon cayenne pepper
¼ teaspoon pure stevia extract powder (or more—adjust to taste)
fresh ground pepper to taste

Mix the dressing ingredients, pour it over the slaw ingredients, mix well, chill, and then serve. Simple and delicious.

MAKES 2 LARGE SERVINGS

Calories: 5 • Calories from fat: 0 • Total fat: 0g
Saturated fat: 0g • Trans fat: 0g • Cholesterol: 0mg
Sodium: 10mg • Total Carbohydrate: 1g
Dietary Fiber: 0g • Sugars: 0g • Protein: 0g
Nutritional content may vary depending upon preparation.

"Where's the Beef?" Bul Go Gee

Bul Go Gee is a Korean charbroiled beef dish. This is a vegan version. There are three parts to this dish: the portobellos, the rice, and the spinach.

Portobellos
6–8 large portobello caps thinly sliced (⅛ inch)
2 tablespoons sesame seeds
4 tablespoons sesame oil
¾ cup Bragg's Liquid Aminos
2 tiny scoops pure stevia extract powder (the tiny scoop that
     comes in the KAL brand = ½₄ teaspoon)
3–4 cloves garlic, minced
8 green onions, sliced
¼–½ teaspoon fresh ground pepper

Combine the sliced portobellos in a large Ziploc with remaining ingredients. Marinate the mushrooms for at least 30 minutes, or ideally 3–5 hours.

Rice
2 cups brown rice (always best to plan ahead and soak the rice)
4 cups pure water (a little less if you soak the rice)

Bring the brown rice to a boil in the water. Cover, reduce heat, and simmer for 40 minutes, or until tender (less time if you have soaked the rice).

Spinach
2–3 large bunches whole-leaf spinach (it looks like too much until it
     steams)
Bragg's Liquid Aminos
sesame oil
sesame seeds
fresh ground pepper (optional)

While the rice is cooking, prepare the steamer for the spinach. When the rice is ready, turn it off, leaving it covered. Steam the spinach for about 5 minutes or until limp. Even in a large pot with a steamer, you will have to do two batches. Once the first batch of spinach is steamed, place in a glass serving bowl and while steaming the second batch of spinach, toss the first with 1–2 tablespoons of sesame seeds, 1–2 tablespoons of Bragg's Aminos, and 1–2 tablespoons of sesame oil. Fresh ground black pepper is optional.

Take the portobellos out of the marinade and place them on a broiling rack or in a glass 13 x 9 baking dish. Broil for 5 minutes at the lowest broiler setting. They just need to be warmed.

Place a serving of rice on a plate, top with a serving of spinach and portobello strips. Season with more Bragg's if desired.

MAKES 4–6 MAIN DISH SERVINGS

Calories: 380 • Calories from fat: 80 • Total fat: 9g
Saturated fat: 1.5g • Trans fat: 0g • Cholesterol: 0mg
Sodium: 1400mg • Total Carbohydrate: 65g
Dietary Fiber: 9g • Sugars: 4g • Protein: 18g
Nutritional content may vary depending upon preparation.

Phase Two/Day One

Mexican Sandwich Filling

½ cup shredded carrots
1 cup finely chopped broccoli
1 cup finely chopped cauliflower
5–6 green onions, chopped
2 cloves garlic, minced
2 teaspoons cumin
1½ teaspoons chili powder
fresh cilantro to taste (optional)
1 tablespoon Soymage Parmesan Cheese (optional)

Mix all of the above and toss with ½ cup ranch dressing. (See Vegan Ranch Dressing recipe page 305.)

Garnishes
shredded lettuce
chopped tomato
avocado

Place the filling on a whole-grain sprouted tortilla, or in a romaine leaf topped with shredded lettuce, tomato, and if desired, avocado. Wrap and enjoy. (This recipe can also be used on bread or toast.)

MAKES 3–4 WRAPS

Calories: 110 • Calories from fat: 70 • Total fat: 8g
Saturated fat: 0g • Trans fat: 0g • Cholesterol: 0mg
Sodium: 290mg • Total Carbohydrate: 8g
Dietary Fiber: 3g • Sugars: 2g • Protein: 3g
Nutritional content may vary depending upon preparation.

Romaine with Lemon Dulse Dressing

Used with permission from Hippocrates Health Institute.

4 cups romaine lettuce, broken into bite-sized pieces
¼ cup sliced red onion
¼ cup shredded carrot
½ cup chopped fresh parsley
¼ cup thinly sliced red cabbage

In a mixing bowl combine all of the above.

Dressing

> 3 tablespoons extra virgin olive oil
> 1 clove garlic, minced
> 1 tablespoon fresh lemon juice
> 3 tablespoons dulse flakes
> cayenne to taste
> pure water as needed to blend

Place all of the dressing ingredients into a blender. Blend well and season to taste.

Toss the dressing with the salad mixture until it is well combined, and serve.

MAKES 2 SERVINGS

Calories: 240 • Calories from fat: 190 • Total fat: 22g
Saturated fat: 3g • Trans fat: 0g • Cholesterol: 0mg
Sodium: 45mg • Total Carbohydrate: 10g
Dietary Fiber: 4g • Sugars: 4g • Protein: 3g
Nutritional content may vary depending upon preparation.

Phase Two/Day Two

Cinnamon Buckwheat Cereal

2 cups buckwheat, soaked in pure water 12–24 hours
½ teaspoon cinnamon
½ teaspoon nutmeg
⅛ teaspoon pure stevia extract powder

Drain the soaked buckwheat, place it in a medium-sized glass bowl, and mix in the stevia and spices. Spread on a dehydrator tray with a teflex sheet. Dehydrate for 12–24 hours. Once it is completely dry, put mixture in a jar. Serve with your choice of milk substitute. (This reminds me of my old favorite: Grape Nuts.)

MAKES 4 SERVINGS

Calories: 80 • Calories from fat: 5 • Total fat: 0.5g
Saturated fat: 30g • Trans fat: 0g • Cholesterol: 0mg
Sodium: 17mg • Total Carbohydrate: 17g
Dietary Fiber: 0g • Sugars: 0g • Protein: 2g
Nutritional content may vary depending upon preparation.

Versatile Vegetable Wraps

For the Wraps
Ezekiel Sprouted Grain Tortillas
Food for Life Brown Rice Tortillas (gluten free)
romaine or collard green leaves

For the Spreads
hummus
Vegenaise
guacamole
mashed avocado

For the Fillings

any vegetables (suggestions: avocado slices, tomato wedges, bell pepper slices, hot or banana peppers, onion, scallions, fresh minced garlic, shredded carrot, shredded zucchini or yellow squash, chopped broccoli, mushrooms)

greens (suggestions: romaine, spinach, butter lettuce)

fresh herbs of choice (suggestions: basil, oregano, parsley, dill, cilantro)

sprouts (suggestions: sunflower, pea greens, broccoli, alfalfa, clover, radish, onion)

For the Sauces/Dressings

salsa
Vegan Ranch Dressing
Italian Olive Oil Dressing

For the Seasonings

sea salt   cayenne
garlic powder   chili powder
onion powder   cumin

There is no wrong way to make a wrap. You could prepare a different wrap every day of the week. The wonderful thing is that a wrap makes a satisfying meal that is almost all raw and can be all raw if you choose to use a leaf as your wrap.

Suggested Procedure: Layer the spread on your wrap. Next sprinkle fresh or dried herbs. Fresh minced garlic can be distributed at this point if you like garlic. Then shred your choice of greens on, followed by the selected vegetables. If you are using a sauce/dressing, pour it on and finish by adding desired seasonings. Make sure that you do not fill it so full that it won't hold together.

Experiment and find the best combinations. You don't always have to use a sauce/dressing or seasonings. You will enjoy these so much that you won't miss animal products.

SERVING SIZE: 1 WRAP

Calories: 360 • Calories from fat: 170 • Total fat: 19g*
Saturated fat: 1.5g • Trans fat: 0g • Cholesterol: 0mg
Sodium: 400mg • Total Carbohydrate: 40g
Dietary Fiber: 11g • Sugars: 2g • Protein: 10g
*Fat is from the tortilla, avocado, and vegan ranch dressing
Nutritional content may vary depending upon preparation.

Healthy Lifestyle Ice Cream

What a way to use your over-ripened bananas! Once bananas are too ripe (brown and spotted), peel them and place them in freezer bags. Make sure they are frozen solid (at least twenty-four hours) before you proceed with this recipe.

2 frozen bananas
½ tablespoon raw almond butter (optional, but adds creaminess)
½ teaspoon vanilla (optional)
⅓ cup frozen organic blueberries, cherries, strawberries, or raspberries (optional)

Place the bananas (chopped into several chunks) in a food processor and blend them until they are like soft serve ice cream, with no chunks remaining. Pulse the processor, and open it and scrape the side walls intermittently. You can add the almond butter now. This process makes plain banana ice cream. This is good, but it is even better if you add ⅓ cup of frozen organic blueberries or frozen organic raspberries once the bananas are creamy.

MAKES 1 SERVING

Calories: 290 • Calories from fat: 50 • Total fat: 6g
Saturated fat: 0.5g • Trans fat: 0g • Cholesterol: 0mg
Sodium: 40mg • Total Carbohydrate: 61g
Dietary Fiber: 8g • Sugars: 33g • Protein: 4g
Nutritional content may vary depending upon preparation.

Italian Olive Oil Dressing

1 cup extra virgin olive oil
½ cup Bragg's Raw Apple Cider Vinegar
¼ cup pure water
juice of one organic lemon
4 cloves garlic, minced or pressed
1 teaspoon sea salt
½ teaspoon turmeric (optional—healthy if you like the taste)
dash of cayenne pepper (not much!)
½ teaspoon onion powder

1 teaspoon oregano
2 teaspoons dried basil or 1 tablespoon fresh basil, chopped
2 tablespoons finely chopped fresh parsley
¼ teaspoon dry mustard

Place all ingredients into a jar with a lid. Put the lid on the jar and shake vigorously. Store at room temperature.

MAKES 15 SERVINGS

Calories: 120 • Calories from fat: 110 • Total fat: 13g
Saturated fat: 2g • Trans fat: 0g • Cholesterol: 0mg
Sodium: 130mg • Total Carbohydrate: 1g
Dietary Fiber: 0g • Sugars: 0g • Protein: 0g
Nutritional content may vary depending upon preparation.

Veggie Pesto Pasta

1 pound brown rice pasta

Veggie Topping
olive oil spray
1 large onion, sliced
3 carrots, cut in julienne strips
1 cup cauliflower florets
1 cup broccoli florets
2 cups sliced mushrooms
sea salt to taste

Veggie Pesto Sauce
9 cups fresh broccoli florets and stems
3 cloves garlic, peeled
½ cup extra virgin olive oil
1 teaspoon sea salt
½ to 1 cup of the steaming water (reserved from the broccoli)

For the Topping: Spray a large skillet with extra virgin olive oil and sauté onion, carrots, 1 cup broccoli, and cauliflower until they begin to get tender. Add the sliced mushrooms and salt to taste, cover, and turn to low.

For the Sauce: Blanch 9 cups broccoli in pure water for 4 minutes or until bright green. Place it in the food processor with the garlic, olive oil, salt, and reserved water. Process until smooth.

Place a serving of pasta on each plate, top with a scoop of pesto
sauce, then top with vegetables. Enjoy.

MAKES 6 SERVINGS

Calories: 470 • Calories from fat: 260 • Total fat: 29g
Saturated fat: 4g • Trans fat: 0g • Cholesterol: 0mg
Sodium: 460mg • Total Carbohydrate: 44g
Dietary Fiber: 7g • Sugars: 4g • Protein: 8g
Nutritional content may vary depending upon preparation.

Phase Two/Day Three

Meatless Cincinnati Chili with Pasta

A vegan version of an old favorite—minus the cheese.

2 cups organic lentils
16-ounce bag of organic kidney beans
3 cups water
2 large onions, chopped
2 cloves garlic, minced
2 tablespoons chili powder
1 teaspoon cinnamon
1 teaspoon cumin
1 teaspoon black pepper
½ teaspoon cayenne pepper
1 teaspoon sea salt
1½ teaspoons allspice
1½ tablespoons raw apple cider vinegar
3 whole bay leaves
1 recipe of Tomato Paste
Whole-grain spaghetti, cooked according to package directions
1 medium onion, chopped (to be left uncooked for use as a topping on each serving, if desired)

Soak lentils and kidney beans in pure water overnight. Drain the lentils and beans, and cover each with pure water in separate pans. Bring each to a boil and simmer until tender. Drain in a colander.

Put all ingredients (except the pasta and extra onion) in a large pot. Bring to a boil. Simmer for three hours. (You can leave it in a Crock Pot on low for longer.) When ready to serve, boil whole grain spaghetti and serve the Cincinnati Chili over the pasta. Top with raw, chopped onions if desired.

MAKES 8–10 SERVINGS

Calories: 430 • Calories from fat: 10 • Total fat: 1.5g
Saturated fat: 0g • Trans fat: 0g • Cholesterol: 0mg
Sodium: 360mg • Total Carbohydrate: 81g
Dietary Fiber: 25g • Sugars: 8g • Protein: 26g
Nutritional content may vary depending upon preparation.

Tomato Paste

Many recipes call for tomato paste. When it comes to health, using tomatoes out of a can is not a good idea. Aluminum or steel cans are not a good idea for any product, much less acidic tomatoes.

This tomato paste recipe is relatively easy. You can make several batches and keep some in your freezer so that it will be handy when you need it. Since it is prepared from whole, organic foods, it is much healthier than canned tomato paste.

> 1 cup diced fresh organic tomatoes (about 2 medium)
> ¼ cup chopped onion
> ⅛ teaspoon dried oregano (or several fresh leaves)
> ¼ teaspoon dried basil (or 4–5 large fresh leaves)
> 1 cup shredded carrot
> 1–2 dates
> sea salt to taste
> 1–2 teaspoons arrowroot powder

Place all ingredients except the arrowroot powder in the blender. Mix well until smooth. Add 1 teaspoon of arrowroot powder, bring this to a boil, reduce heat, and simmer until thickened, stirring occasionally. If it does not get thick enough for your recipe, add the second teaspoon of arrowroot powder.

Use right away, or store in the freezer. You can freeze this in glass jars as long as you leave about an inch of space at the top and do not put the lid on too tight.

MAKES 8–10 SERVINGS

Calories: 30 • Calories from fat: 0 • Total fat: 0g
Saturated fat: 0g • Trans fat: 0g • Cholesterol: 0mg
Sodium: 10mg • Total Carbohydrate: 8g
Dietary Fiber: 1g • Sugars: 5g • Protein: 1g
Nutritional content may vary depending upon preparation.

Favorite Tropical Smoothie

½ mango, cut into chunks
¼–½ fresh pineapple with juice
1 orange, juiced with a citrus juicer
1 large or 2 small frozen bananas, broken into several pieces
½ cup frozen organic cherries or blueberries
2 tablespoons ground flaxseed

Place the mango and pineapple into a blender with the juice from the pineapple and the fresh-squeezed orange juice. Process until smooth. Add the frozen banana and cherries or berries. Process again until smooth and thick. If it gets too thick, you can add a small amount of cold pure water. Once it is processed, add the ground flaxseed and pulse again to mix well.

MAKES 2 SERVINGS

Calories: 320 • Calories from fat: 45 • Total fat: 4.5g
Saturated fat: 0.5g • Trans fat: 0g • Cholesterol: 0mg
Sodium: 10mg • Total Carbohydrate: 73g
Dietary Fiber: 10g • Sugars: 45g • Protein: 5g
Nutritional content may vary depending upon preparation.

Banana Nut and Seed Bars

1 large or 2 small bananas, mashed
1 teaspoon vanilla
½ cup raisins (optional)
½ cup raw sunflower seeds
¾ cup raw walnuts
½ cup raw pumpkin seeds
1 tablespoon whole flaxseeds
1 tablespoon ground flaxseeds
¼ cup sesame seeds
¾ cup raw macadamia nuts
1 cup raw almonds
½ teaspoon sea salt
¼–½ cup honey (whatever amount is needed to enable you to mix it
    all together)

Combine ingredients. Mix well, adding just enough honey to hold it together. The amount will vary depending on the size of the bananas. Spread onto a teflex dehydrator sheet and dehydrate at 105°F for 6 hours. Place another dehydrator tray without a teflex sheet on top of this one. Flip over and peel the teflex sheet off and score with a pizza cutter. Dehydrate until desired texture: you can let it dehydrate for a shorter time for chewy bars or longer for a crunchy consistency.

MAKES 25 SERVINGS

Calories: 66 • Calories from fat: 44 • Total fat: 5g
Saturated fat: 0.5g • Trans fat: 0g • Cholesterol: 0mg
Sodium: 24mg • Total Carbohydrate: 4.5g
Dietary Fiber: 1g • Sugars: 2.5g • Protein: 2g
Nutritional content may vary depending upon preparation.

Spicy Raw Nuts

These nuts taste like you cooked them, yet they still have the healthful enzymes.

Soak selected nuts overnight in pure water. (You may use raw almonds, pecans, walnuts, Brazil, pistachios, or hazelnuts. You may choose one kind of nut or a variety of the above.)

Drain the water. Place the drained nuts in a bowl. Sprinkle with a small amount of Bragg's Liquid Aminos and then with any of the following:

> cayenne (for extra health benefits and spiciness)
> garlic powder
> onion powder
> chili powder
> cumin powder
> Frontier Italian Seasoning
> ground flaxseed

To make the spicy nuts Mexican flavored, season with chili powder, cumin, onion, and garlic. For Italian-flavored nuts, use Italian Seasoning, onion, and garlic. Adding ground flaxseed with the seasonings helps them to adhere to the nuts.

Mix well and place the spiced nuts in a single layer on your dehydrator tray. Put them in the dehydrator at 105°F for 24–48 hours. Larger nuts, such as Brazil nuts, usually take longer to dehydrate.

SERVING SIZE ¼ CUP

Calories: 250 • Calories from fat: 180 • Total fat: 19g
Saturated fat: 3.5g • Trans fat: 0g • Cholesterol: 0mg
Sodium: 45mg • Total Carbohydrate: 14g
Dietary Fiber: 2g • Sugars: 3g • Protein: 8g
Nutritional content may vary depending upon preparation.

Yellow Squash Carrot Salad

From Hippocrates' kitchen.

> 1 yellow summer squash, julienned
> ½ carrot, julienned
> ½ cup chopped fresh parsley
> ¼ red onion, julienned
> 1 teaspoon dried oregano
> 1 clove garlic, minced
> 1½ tablespoons extra virgin olive oil
> 1 teaspoon fresh lemon juice
> ½ teaspoon ground cumin

In a mixing bowl, combine all ingredients. Mix well and season to taste with dulse or kelp powder or Bragg's Liquid Aminos.

MAKES 2 SERVINGS

Calories: 170 • Calories from fat: 100 • Total fat: 11g
Saturated fat: 1.5g • Trans fat: 0g • Cholesterol: 0mg
Sodium: 20mg • Total Carbohydrate: 18g
Dietary Fiber: 5g • Sugars: 6g • Protein: 3g
Nutritional content may vary depending upon preparation.

Phase Three/All-Raw Day

Uncooked Whole-Grain Buckwheat Breakfast

Buckwheat soaked overnight is soft and ready to eat. It does not require cooking, the enzymes are still intact, and it is just as easy as opening a box of cereal, yet the health benefits are much increased.

Soak ½ cup of buckwheat overnight in 1 cup of pure water.

In the morning, pour it through a strainer to drain if any water remains (it should be nearly all absorbed), rinse it, and place it in a bowl. Sprinkle with stevia, cinnamon, and nutmeg. Add a small amount of milk alternative, if desired, and enjoy.

MAKES 1 SERVING

Calories: 420 • Calories from fat: 20 • Total fat: 2g
Saturated fat: 0g • Trans fat: 0g • Cholesterol: 0mg
Sodium: 5mg • Total Carbohydrate: 87g
Dietary Fiber: 1g • Sugars: 0g • Protein: 12g
Nutritional content may vary depending upon preparation.

Veggie Flax Crackers

Soak 1½ cups of flaxseed in 3 cups of water for at least 3 hours or overnight.

Drain the flaxseed using a strainer and stirring with a spoon.

In a bowl, combine the flaxseed with:

> dash of cayenne
> 1 tablespoon chili powder
> 2 teaspoons cumin powder
> ½ medium-sized onion, finely chopped

½ large carrot, shredded
1 large clove garlic, minced
2 tablespoons flaxseed, ground
½ teaspoon sea salt
½ teaspoon garlic powder

Spread the mixture over two dehydrator trays lined with teflex sheets. It should be spread in a thin layer, just covering the sheet without gaps. Dehydrate for an hour, then score it into squares with a pizza cutter and continue to dehydrate overnight or all day. Then turn onto another tray without a teflex sheet and peel off the sheet. Dehydrate until dried and crispy (another 12–24 hours). The result will be a crispy, spicy cracker that is good for dipping in salsa or eating plain.

MAKES 40 SERVINGS

Calories: 17 • Calories from fat: 12 • Total fat: 1g
Saturated fat: 0g • Trans fat: 0g • Cholesterol: 0mg
Sodium: 11mg • Total Carbohydrate: 1g
Dietary Fiber: 0.5g • Sugars: 0.1g • Protein: 0.5g
Nutritional content may vary depending upon preparation.

Mexican Cabbage Salad

From Ken Blue

6 cups cabbage, chopped or coarsely shredded (1 small cabbage)
5 scallions, washed and diced
1 tablespoon fresh cilantro, chopped
1 recipe Walnut Taco Filling (about three cups) (recipe on
    page 326)

Toss first three ingredients with ¼ cup Basic Dressing (recipe follows) in a medium-sized bowl. Refrigerate to "marinate" until you are ready to serve. Add the Walnut Taco Filling and mix well just prior to serving.

MAKES 4–6 SERVINGS

Calories: 480 • Calories from fat: 390 • Total fat: 43g
Saturated fat: 3g • Trans fat: 0g • Cholesterol: 0mg
Sodium: 190mg • Total Carbohydrate: 14g
Dietary Fiber: 7g • Sugars: 3g • Protein: 17g

Basic Dressing

¼ cup fresh lime (or lemon) juice
1 teaspoon kelp powder
¼ cup olive oil
1 large clove garlic, minced
dash of cayenne

Place all of the ingredients in a blender and blend on high until well mixed. Reserve the extra dressing for use on another salad. You can add herbs to season.

Calories: 270 • Calories from fat: 250 • Total fat: 28g
Saturated fat: 4g • Trans fat: 0g • Cholesterol: 0mg
Sodium: 0mg • Total Carbohydrate: 4g
Dietary Fiber: 1g • Sugars: 1g • Protein: 0g
Nutritional content may vary depending upon preparation.

Quick and Easy Walnut Taco Filling

From Ken Blue

>   3 cups walnuts
>   ½ teaspoon garlic powder
>   2 tablespoons plus 1 teaspoon chili powder
>   ⅛ teaspoon cayenne
>   ½ teaspoon cumin powder
>   3 teaspoons Bragg's Liquid Aminos

In a food processor, combine all ingredients except the Bragg's Aminos. Pulse lightly while adding the Aminos.

This can be used in a romaine leaf with taco toppings to make a delicious "taco" or to replace the meat in your taco salad.

MAKES 6–8 HALF-CUP SERVINGS

Calories: 400 • Calories from fat: 340 • Total fat: 37g
Saturated fat: 2g • Trans fat: 0g • Cholesterol: 0mg
Sodium: 180mg • Total Carbohydrate: 8g
Dietary Fiber: 5g • Sugars: 1g • Protein: 16g
Nutritional content may vary depending upon preparation.

Tantalizing Trio

From Ken Blue

A legitimate treat for the sweet tooth—salad that tastes like dessert. Many people do not realize that you can eat sweet potatoes and butternut squash uncooked. This delicious, enzyme-active recipe is a treat everyone will enjoy.

Salad
1 medium-sized butternut squash, peeled, seeded, and thinly sliced
   in a food processor
1 medium-sized sweet potato, organic and unpeeled, thinly sliced
   in a food processor
1 large carrot, organic, unpeeled, thinly sliced in a food processor

Dressing
¾ cup (or 6 ounces) chopped carrot
⅛ cup fresh lemon juice
½ cup raw, organic sesame oil
¾ teaspoon fresh ginger, minced
¾ teaspoon kelp powder
1 teaspoon cinnamon
¾ teaspoon pumpkin pie spice
½ tiny scoop stevia
1 tablespoon Frontier vanilla (without alcohol)

Combine salad ingredients in a medium sized bowl.

In a Vita Mix (or good blender), mix the dressing ingredients.

(If you do not have a Vita Mix, this dressing may require that the carrot be shredded before blending to ensure that the result is a smooth dressing.)

Use just enough of the dressing to coat the vegetables well. You may need all of it or just most of it depending upon the size of your butternut squash and sweet potato. Serve immediately or chill and serve.

MAKES 4–6 SERVINGS

Calories: 240 • Calories from fat: 170 • Total fat: 19g
Saturated fat: 2.5g • Trans fat: 0g • Cholesterol: 0mg
Sodium: 35mg • Total Carbohydrate: 18g
Dietary Fiber: 3g • Sugars: 4g • Protein: 1g
Nutritional content may vary depending upon preparation.

Brazil Nut Loaf, Paté, or Crackers

From Ken Blue

> 2 cups Brazil nuts, soaked in water
> 1 cup roughly chopped carrot
> ¼ cup chopped red onion
> 2 stalks celery, chopped
> 1 clove garlic, peeled
> 1½ teaspoons caraway seed
> 1 teaspoon fennel seed
> 1 teaspoon onion powder
> 2 teaspoons Bragg's Liquid Aminos
>
> **Optional Stir-Ins**
> ½ cup chopped fresh parsley or dill
> ¼ cup finely diced onion
> ¼ cup finely diced celery

In a food processor, process all of the above, except the liquid aminos, until smooth. If you have a juicer with a blank screen, a smoother mixture can be acquired by processing the mixture with this homogenizing attachment. Once it is processed, you can stir in the liquid aminos to taste along with the optional stir-ins, if desired.

This can be served as paté, rolled in a leaf of romaine with green onion or other veggies, or formed into a loaf (1-inch thick and oblong) and placed in the dehydrator at 105°F until it is warm (3–5 hours).

This recipe can be eaten as a paté for one meal, and the leftovers can be spread out over a teflex sheet on a dehydrator tray to a thickness of ⅛ inch. Score and dehydrate until it is crunchy like a cracker for a great snack.

MAKES 8 SERVINGS

Calories: 200 • Calories from fat: 170 • Total fat: 19g
Saturated fat: 4.5g • Trans fat: 0g • Cholesterol: 0mg
Sodium: 75mg • Total Carbohydrate: 6g
Dietary Fiber: 3g • Sugars: 2g • Protein: 5g
Nutritional content may vary depending upon preparation.

Kitchen Essentials

Since you are embarking on a new lifestyle, you will have to stock your kitchen with new staples. No longer will white sugar, brown sugar, enriched wheat flour, shortening, vegetable oil, milk, cheese, and white rice be staples. Below is a list of kitchen equipment and staple foods that you will find helpful for the *NBFA* Lifestyle. You need not rush and purchase all of these things immediately. In transition, purchase a few items at a time until you have your kitchen furnished and equipped to suit your new lifestyle.

Kitchen Gadgets

Garlic Press. Since garlic is a healing food with natural antioxidant properties and other health benefits, it is a regular part of a healthy diet. A press makes garlic use so much simpler. There are even presses that do not require you to peel the garlic.

Olive Oil Spritzing Spray Bottle. Store-bought cooking sprays have unhealthy additives. High-quality organic olive oil can be used as a spray for cooking when you purchase a bottle that is filled with your own oil. You simply pump and spray. Much less oil is required when you use this gadget. You can mist healthy oil on your salads and avoid a puddle on the plate. The mist sticks to the vegetables. Warm, drained pasta can be misted and then eaten with steamed vegetables and seasonings. This beats cooking with the oil.

Salad Spinner. This is perfect for preparing washed greens for a salad. They are easily dried, crispy (especially if you spin and refrigerate while you prepare the other vegetables), and ready for use.

Food Processor. An essential tool for many recipes: sauces, hummus, crackers, ice cream, and so on.

Blender. A must for smoothie preparation and very helpful for salad dressings and other sauces (see Appendix D for recommendations).

Coffee Grinder. For use in grinding flaxseeds.

Stainless Steel Strainer.

Nut Milk Bag. A must for making rice, seed, or nut milk. Either a nut milk bag or a piece of cloth is necessary for straining the milk before use.

Excalibur Dehydrator (optional, but very helpful). While not an essential, a dehydrator is helpful for preparing raw crackers, and raw, soaked, dehydrated, and seasoned or plain nuts and seeds. This particular dehydrator is recommended because it has a temperature control to regulate the temperature as low as 95°F to preserve enzymes.

Champion or Green Star Juicer (optional). Not only is it great to have access to fresh vegetable juices, it is also perfect for making nut butters and ice cream. Green Star is actually our choice for juicing greens.

Handheld Citrus/Lemon Squeezer. Lemon juice is an ingredient in many of the recipes, so having a small citrus-squeezing device is quite convenient. Processed lemon juice is not organic and has other additives.

Glass Kitchenware. Use glass whenever possible to replace plastic bowls, dishes, and cups, and metal/aluminum baking sheets.

Baking Stones. Use these to replace metal baking sheets (which usually contain aluminum).

Steaming Basket. To fit into a covered pan for steaming vegetables.

Parchment Paper. Use this instead of foil, which leaches aluminum into your food.

Food Items

Whole Grains

amaranth	oats
brown rice	quinoa
buckwheat	teff
millet	wheat, spelt, or kamut berries

Oils

extra virgin olive oil (Beyond Health Extra Virgin Olive Oil)
flaxseed oil (refrigerated)
hempseed oil (refrigerated)
raw virgin coconut oil (Beyond Health Extra Virgin Coconut Oil)

Nuts and Seeds (all raw and organic)

almonds	pecans
Brazil nuts	pistachios
flaxseed	pumpkin seeds
hazelnuts	sesame seeds
hempseed	sunflower seeds
macadamia nuts	walnuts

Sea Vegetables

Sea vegetables are exceptionally high in mineral content along with vitamins. They are an asset to any diet. We have provided a few recipes that call for sea vegetables so that you can experiment with them. If you don't like them at first, don't give up. Try again because they will grow on you.

Arame
Dulse (You can make this into a naturally salty, crunchy "chip" by soaking/dehydrating.)
Dulse flakes
Hijiki
Kelp powder (This can be found at most health stores and is an easy way to increase minerals in your diet and replace salt in recipes.)

Pantry Items

These can all be found in health-food stores.

Kelp and/or dulse powder. Since they are naturally salty, the flakes from dulse and kelp can be used in place of salt to add saltiness and mineral content to dishes without giving the recipes a high sodium content.

Celtic sea salt. Sun dried and without anticaking agents, if possible.

Stevia extract powder. See Appendix D for recommendations.

Bragg's Raw Apple Cider Vinegar.

Bragg's Liquid Aminos. Use in place of soy sauce or just to add saltiness without salt.

Arrowroot Powder. For thickening—use in the same quantity instead of corn starch.

Raw tahini.

Xanthan gum. For use in gluten-free baking.

Better Choices for Processed Foods

These can be found in health-food stores.

Edward and Sons Baked Brown Rice Crackers with no added oils

Mary's Gone Crackers

Ezekiel Sprouted Grain Tortillas

Food for Life Brown Rice Tortillas

Healthy Hemp Tortillas by French Meadow Bakery

Sunshine Burgers. A decent health-food store veggie burger without preservatives.

Tinkyada Brown Rice Pasta. This brand tastes the most like ordinary pasta and cooks without becoming mushy or starchy.

Soymage Parmesan*

Follow Your Heart Vegenaise* (grapeseed oil variety). This can replace mayonnaise at the start, but should not figure prominently in your diet on a daily basis. For special occasions only.

Organic spaghetti sauces sold in glass jars. Look for varieties with all organic ingredients and no added sugar, sweeteners, or poor-quality oils.

Salsa. Look for brands, such as Drew's, that incorporate all organic vegetables and no sugar or sweeteners.

*Use as a transition item.

When it comes to store-bought salad dressings, we have been unable to find a truly healthy variety due to the fact that poor-quality oils, various vinegars, and sweeteners are used in most commercially prepared dressings. Homemade dressings provide the best option. When you have a day off, simply prepare enough dressing for the week ahead so that it is readily available.

Ready . . . Set . . . Change!

The steps and menus outlined in this chapter illustrate how to live this lifestyle, and they are optional. Ultimately, you have to make the *NBFA* Lifestyle *your own* in a way that works for your situation. People are not cookie-cutter images. Rather, we are all individuals, and we don't want you to try to force yourself into a plan that does not work for you. Using the wealth of information, menu plans, and recipes as a blueprint, begin to change your habits along all Six Pathways so that you are overcoming deficiency and avoiding toxicity— the two causes of overweight. Experiment until you find exercise workouts and meals that you enjoy and that fit your unique circumstances. Since this is not a temporary change, but a lifestyle, it must be tailored (while your mind-set is also altered) so that it is comfortable for you and one that you can live with permanently.

Appendix A

Beyond Health

After my near-death experience and learning what I had to learn in order to recover my health, I decided in 1991 to devote the remainder of my life to helping others to get healthy and stay healthy in order to end the epidemic of chronic and degenerative disease in America. To achieve this, I started a company called Beyond Health, whose purpose is to provide ongoing health education along with access to the highest-quality health-supporting products on the market.

Beyond Health supplies an educational tool called the Beyond Health Model™. This is a model of health based on the concept of One Disease, Two Causes, and Six Pathways. The model is so simple, yet it is so powerful that it revolutionizes our understanding of health and disease. Many people have been able to heal themselves of seemingly incurable, even fatal diseases by moving themselves in the right direction on the Six Pathways. A free report outlining and explaining the Beyond Health Model is available at www.beyondhealth.com.

Another educational service is the Beyond Health Radio Show. This weekly talk show delivers the latest and most highly advanced health information available anywhere. It is available live in selected cities as well as 24/7 online at www.beyondhealth.com.

We also publish *Beyond Health News,* a bimonthly newsletter filled with information that is decades ahead of the mainstream media. It cuts through the contradictions and confusion, translating a chaotic mountain of medical and scientific data into the critical knowledge that people *must* have in order maintain healthy bodies. *Beyond Health News* is available in print and online. For additional information and subscriptions, go to the Beyond Health website or call 800-250-3063.

Beyond Health is a supplier of the highest-quality health-supporting supplements and products on the market. There is an enormous amount of conflicting information regarding the selection of vitamin supplements and other health products. Consumers remain confused about how to make the best choices. It is difficult to know, merely by reading the label, if products are healthy or toxic or whether they will do what you want them to do. Even small amounts of impurities and toxins in supplements are sufficient to harm your health. *Beyond Health researches and approves only the safest and most effective choices in supplements, foods, and personal products*—discerning between those that claim to be the best and those for which there is credible evidence that they really are the best. For example, it took eighteen months of study and analysis to find a brand of toothpaste that did not contain toxic ingredients but still cleaned teeth well. It took two years to find a safe and effective deodorant. It took eight months to find a pure and healthy brand of olive oil. Vitamin supplements were the biggest challenge. Almost half of all vitamin brands do not dissolve quickly enough to be of use to the human body. Many do not contain all the nutrients listed on the label. Most brands contain cheap ingredients that have only marginal biological activity, and some of these ingredients can be harmful. *The most expensive vitamin pill in the world is one that doesn't work.* For these reasons, Beyond Health puts its own brand on a limited number of products to assure consumers that these meet the highest standards of quality and effectiveness. Beyond Health is the number-one premium health brand in America.

Selecting safe and effective products is a difficult, time-consuming and unique service. Take advantage of this service, and obtain the safest and most effective products for yourself and family. Contact Beyond Health at www.beyondhealth.com or at 800-250-3063.

Appendix B

The Never Be Fat Again *Tracking Journal*

*If other people can make significant changes, why not you?
Remember, nothing will change until you do. Embrace change
as a positive catalyst, one that will give you more freedom and
peace of mind. If you keep on doing what you've always done,
you'll keep on getting what you've always got.*

—Jack Canfield

With the information and the tools in this book, you *can*
make a dramatic difference in your health and your life. Use
this journal as your week-by-week guide to keep you on track
along your transformation to health. You can photocopy the
pages and fill them in as you need them.

Date I Began the *Never Be Fat Again* Lifestyle: _____

Health Issues Before Beginning:

Beginning Weight: _____

My Realistic Goal Weight:_____

My Starting
Measurements: Chest:_____   Waist: _____ Hips:_____

            Upper
            Arm: _____   Thigh: _____ Calf: _____
                                (thickest part)

Spend some time reflecting on your life and what you want it to be in every realm. Set clearly definable and realistic goals for yourself for each pathway. We recommend you insert one page behind this page for each pathway—Nutrition, Toxin, Mental, Physical, Genetic, and Medical. Begin by listing at least one goal for each pathway. As you read this book and incorporate the lifestyle, you will most likely want to add new goals for each aspect of your life.

The one thing that separates winners from losers is, WIN-NERS TAKE ACTION!

—Anthony Robbins

Appendix C

Never Be Fat Again *Daily Accountability*

(COPY THESE PAGES AND FILL IN AS NEEDED.)

Day/Date: _____ Weekly weight: _____

Pounds lost: Week _____ Total _____

Last night I went to bed at: _____ Morning urine pH: ____
Affirmations: _____

Today I arose at: _____ Hours slept: _____

Breathing exercises: AM ____ PM____

Minutes of sunshine: Minutes of reading: _____

Water consumption (check off amount consumed):
8   8   8   8   8   8   8   8 (/ for 4 oz. X for 8 oz)

Exercise/Activity (type, duration, and time of day):

Food consumption (list the time when you ate and whether you were hungry):

Breakfast:

341

Lunch:

Supper:

Snacks:

Supplements:

Evaluation/response to foods eaten:

Estimated percentage of raw foods eaten today: _____% (by weight)
_____ servings of vegetables today
_____ servings of fruit today
Elimination (list times of bowel movements): _____
Food cravings and times:
Positive and negative feelings after eating (food eaten/physical and emotional response):

Things I will do better tomorrow:

Rate from 1–10 (10 being the highest)
Energy level: Positive attitude:

Stress level: Overeating:

Inspiring quotes/Things to remember:

Appendix D

Product Recommendations

Throughout this book, references have been made to various products, including:

Acid/Alkaline	Saunas
pH Testing Paper	Shower Filters
Blenders	Skin Treatments
Carpet Cleaning Products	Stevia
Coconut Oil	Sugar Substitutes
Insecticides	Vitamin/Mineral
Olive Oil	Supplements
Rebounders	Water Purifiers

Because companies are bought and sold and product quality can change, we recommend you call Beyond Health at 800-250-3063 to get the latest recommendations for the highest-quality choices.

Products for Weight Loss

Following is a list of supplements that we recommend for a weight-loss program:

A multivitamin/mineral formula (Beyond Health Multi Vit/Min)
A high-quality vitamin C (Beyond Health Vit-C)
Detoxification support (Beyond Health Cellular Detox Formula)
Cellular repair nutrients (Beyond Health Cellular Repair Formula)

Minerals for bone support (Beyond Health Bone Support
    Formula)
Essential fatty acids (Beyond Health EFA Formula, Beyond
    Health Coconut Oil, Beyond Health Olive Oil, Barlean's
    Flax Oil, Carlson Cod Liver Oil)
Acetyl-L-Carnitine
Vitamin E
Vitamin B_{12} and folic acid (Perque Vessel Health Guard)
Dietary fiber (Perque Regularity Guard)
Coenzyme Q_{10} (Perque Mito Guard)
L-glutamine (Perque Endura Pak Guard)
Lipoic acid and N-acetyl-L-cysteine (ThioDox)

Products for pH Balance
Magnesium Plus
Choline Citrate
pH Paper

For assistance with the above, call Beyond Health for a free
consultation with a nutritional counselor: 800-250-3063.

Appendix E

Recommended Reading

If you have not yet read *Never Be Sick Again* by Raymond Francis, that is our first suggestion. Other recommended books include:

Health and Nutrition Secrets That Can Save Your Life by Dr. Russell Blaylock

Natural Strategies for Cancer Patients by Dr. Russell Blaylock

Excitotoxins by Dr. Russell Blaylock

Love, Medicine and Miracles by Dr. Bernie Siegal

Eat to Live by Joel Fuhrman

The China Study by Dr. T. Colin Campbell

Toxic Overload by Dr. Paula Baillie-Hamilton

Fit for Life Not Fat for Life by Harvey Diamond

The Power of Focus by Jack Canfield, Mark Victor Hansen, and Les Hewitt

Your Best Life Now by Joel Osteen

The Sprouting Book by Ann Wigmore

Don't Drink Your Milk! by Dr. Frank Oski

Lick the Sugar Habit by Nancy Appleton

A Cancer Battle Plan by Ann Frahm

God's Way to Ultimate Health by Dr. George Malkmus

Living Foods for Optimum Health by Dr. Brian Clement

Breaking the Food Seduction by Dr. Neal Barnard

Appendix F

We've Made It Easy for You to Never Be Fat Again

Get a free online lesson now! Find out how simple it can be to achieve a healthier, slimmer you.

- We've created a day-by-day, step-by-step interactive multimedia experience that walks you through creating your daily plan for lifelong *Never Be Fat Again* results!
- Each fun daily lesson takes just a couple of minutes.
- For the price of a cup of tea per day, you can achieve your dream of normal weight.

The advanced science of *Never Be Fat Again* is the most comprehensive weight-loss program ever presented, but we've done all the hard work for you. We've taken the most important information out of the book and the key action items, and we present them to you in an entertaining, educational, and *easy-to-do* format that will put you on the path to lifelong healthy weight. We have reduced this to quick three- to ten-minute overviews on each topic in the book. It's laid out in thirteen fun and exciting lessons that take only a few minutes each day.

Once you've completed all the multimedia programs and worksheets, you'll have your daily plan that makes it easy for you to achieve your goals, effortlessly and easily.

Now, close your eyes for a moment. . . . Imagine your perfect healthy body. . . . Imagine having and maintaining that healthy weight for the rest of your life. That's what we will help you achieve! Now that you understand how it works through reading the book, the multimedia education will motivate you and provide a specific customized daily plan, making it easy for you to follow.

Go to www.nbfamadeeasy.com now and we'll give you the first lesson FREE. With that alone, you'll be on the path to finally achieving your healthy lifelong weight. Start today and make this the very first day that you make that change that will truly last. (You're just moments away from getting instant access.)

Bibliography

Anderson, Rosalind. (1995). "Toxic Emissions from Carpets." *Journal of Nutritional and Environmental Medicine* 5, 375–86.

Aronne, L. J., et al. (2001, August 15). "Intervening in the Obesity Epidemic." *Patient Care,* 92–106.

Atkins, Robert C. (2002). *Dr. Atkins' New Diet Revolution.* New York: Avon Books, HarperCollins Publishers.

Baillie-Hamilton, Paula. (2002, November 2). "Chemical Toxins: A Hypothesis to Explain the Global Obesity Epidemic." *Journal of Alternative and Complimentary Medicine,* 185–92.

———. (2005). *Toxic Overload.* New York: Avery, Penguin Group, Inc.

Balch, James F., and Phyllis A. Balch. (2000). *Prescription for Nutritional Healing.* New York: Avery, Penguin Putnam Inc.

Barnard, Neal D. (2001, Spring). "Turn Off the Fat Genes." *Good Medicine,* 12–13.

Barnard, Neal D., et al. (2005, September). "The Effects of a Low-Fat, Plant-Based Dietary Intervention on Body Weight, Metabolism, and Insulin Sensitivity." *The American Journal of Medicine,* 991–97.

Beasley, Joseph D., and Jerry J. Swift. (1989). *The Kellogg Report.* Annandale-on-Hudson, NY: The Institute of Health Policy and Practice.

Beecher, Henry K. (1959). "The Powerful Placebo." *Journal of the American Medical Association* 159, 1602–6.

Blair, Steven N., and Tom S. Church. (2004, September 8). "The Fitness, Obesity, and Health Equation." *Journal of the American Medical Association,* 1232–34.

Blaylock, Russell L. (1997). *Excitotoxins.* Santa Fe, NM: Health Press.

———. (2002). *Health and Nutrition Secrets.* Albuquerque, NM: Health Press.

———. (2003). *Natural Strategies for Cancer Patients.* New York: Kensington Publishing Corp.

Bourne, J. R. (2004). "Roles of Unsaturated Fatty Acids (Especially Omega-3 Fatty Acids) in the Brain at Various Stages of Aging." *Journal of Nutritional Health and Aging* 8(3), 163–74.

Bragg, Paul C., and Patricia Bragg. (2006). *Apple Cider Vinegar Miracle Health System,* 54th Edition. Santa Barbara, CA: Health Science.

349

————. (2004). *Bragg Healthy Lifestyle*. Santa Barbara, CA: Health Science.

Bunyan, J., et al. (1976). "The Induction of Obesity in Rodents by Means of Monosodium Glutamate." *British Journal of Nutrition* 35, 25–39.

Caccamese, S.M., et al. (2002, June). "Comparing Patient and Physician Perception of Weight Status with Body Mass Index." *American Journal of Medicine* 112, 6662–66.

Campbell, T. Colin. (2005). *The China Study*. Dallas: BenBella Books.

Canfield, Jack, Mark Victor Hansen, and Les Hewitt. (2000). *The Power of Focus*. Deerfield Beach, FL: Health Communications, Inc.

Chen, Ling, et al. (2005). "Hyperglycemia Inhibits the Uptake of Dehydroascorbate in Tubular Epithelial Cell." *American Journal of Nephrology* 25, 459–65.

Colbert, Don. (2001). *Toxic Relief*. Lake Mary, FL: Siloam Publishing, A Strang Company.

Collantes, Rochelle, et al. (2004, August). "Nonalcoholic Fatty Liver Disease and the Epidemic of Obesity." *Cleveland Clinic Journal of Medicine*, 657–64.

Cortlandt Forum. (2004, April). "Atkins Diet Raises Concerns," 22.

Crossing the Quality Chasm: A New Health System for the 21st Century. (2001). Washington, DC: National Academy Press.

Dansinger, M. L., et al. (2005, January 5). "Comparison of the Atkins, Ornish, Weight Watchers, and Zone Diets for Weight Loss and Heart Disease Risk Reduction." *Journal of the American Medical Association*, 43–53.

Davidson, M. H., et al. (1999). "Comparison of the Effects of Lean Red Meat vs. Lean White Meat on Serum Lipid Levels among Free-living Persons with Hypercholesterolemia: A Long-term Randomized Clinical Trial." *Archives of Internal Medicine* 159(12), 1331–38.

Day, Lorraine. (1997). *You Can't Improve on God*. Thousand Palms, CA: Rockford Press.

Dennison, B. A. (1996). "Fruit Juice Consumption by Infants and Children: A Review." *Journal of the American College of Nutrition* 15(5), 4–11S.

Diamond, Harvey. (2000). *Fit for Life, A New Beginning*. New York: Kensington Publishing Corp.

————. (2003). *Fit for Life, Not Fat for Life*. Deerfield Beach, FL: Health Communications.

Diamond, Marilyn. (1990). *The American Vegetarian Cookbook from the Fit for Life Kitchen*. New York: Warner Books.

Dufty, William. (1986, reissue edition). *Sugar Blues*. New York: Warner Books.

Erasmus, Udo. (1986). *Fats and Oils*. Vancouver, Canada: Alive Books.

Ershoff, B. H. (1976). "Synergistic Toxicity of Food Additives in Rats Fed a Diet Low in Fiber." *Journal of Food Science* 41, 949–51.

Fife, Bruce. (2002). *Eat Fat, Look Thin.* Colorado Springs: Piccadilly Books.

Fontaine, K. R., et al. (2003). "Years of Life Lost Due to Obesity." *Journal of the American Medical Association* 289, 187–93.

Foster, G. D., et al. (2003). "A Randomized Trial of a Low Carbohydrate Diet for Obesity." *New England Journal of Medicine* 348, 2082–90.

Francis, Raymond. (2002). *Never Be Sick Again.* Deerfield Beach, FL: Health Communications.

———. (2002, January/February). "Bouncing Magic." *Beyond Health News,* 4–5.

———. (2004, March/April). "Understanding Disease." *Beyond Health News,* 4–5.

Friedman, J. M. (2000, April 6). "Obesity in the New Millennium." *Nature,* 632–34.

Furhman, Joel. (2003). *Eat to Live.* New York: Little Brown and Company.

Gallo, Roe. (2001, December 25). *Perfect Body.* Ashland, OR: Jack Johnston Seminars.

Gillman, Matthew W., et al. (2001, May 16). "Risk of Overweight Among Adolescents Who Were Breastfed as Infants." *Journal of the American Medical Association,* 2461–67.

Gittleman, Ann Louise. (1996). *Get the Sugar Out.* New York: Three Rivers Press.

Gofman, John. (1999). *Radiation from Medical Procedures in the Pathogenesis of Cancer and Ischemic Heart Disease: Dose Response Studies with Physicians per 100,000 Population.* San Francisco: Committee for Nuclear Responsibility Books.

Good Medicine. (2003, Autumn). "Overweight and Obesity," 5.

Greaser, Jennifer, and John J. Whyte. (2004, September 1). "Childhood Obesity: Is There Effective Treatment?" *Consultant,* 1349–53.

Haas, Elson. (1992). *Staying Healthy with Nutrition.* Berkeley, CA: Celestial Arts Publishing.

Hay, William Howard. (1933). *A New Health Era.* New York: Mount Pocono.

Haupt, K. A. (1982). "Gastrointestinal Factors in Hunger and Satiety." *Neuroscience Biobehavioral Review* 6(2), 145–64.

Henner, Marilu. (1998). *Total Health Makeover.* New York: HarperCollins.

Internal Medicine News. (2000, May 15). "Obesity Stunts Nighttime Blood Pressure Decline," 28.

———. (2003, June 1). "Regular Breakfast May Lower Risk for Obesity," 6.

————. (2003, September 1). "Dieting, Exercise Must Accompany Obesity Drugs," 26.

————. (2003, September 1). "Is Obesity a Disease?" 13.

————. (2004, September 1). "Obesity May Be Cause of Infertility in Men," 36.

Internal Medicine World Report. (2003, September). "British Scientists Discredit Atkins Diet," 4.

————. (2005, January). "Obesity a Risk for Esophageal Cancer," 22.

(2000, November). *Journal of the American College of Cardiology* 36, 1565–71.

Kahn, H. S., et al. (1997). "Stable Behaviors Associated with Adults' 10-Year Change in Body Mass Index and Likelihood of Gain at the Waist." *American Journal of Public Health* 87(5), 747–57.

Katz, David L. (2000). *Nutrition in Clinical Practice.* Philadelphia: Lippincott-Williams & Wilkins.

Kopelman, Peter G. (2000, April 6). "Obesity as a Medical Problem." *Nature,* 635–43.

Lau, Karen, et al. (2006). "Synergistic Interactions Between Commonly Used Food Additives in a Developmental Neurotoxicity Test." *Toxicological Sciences* 90(1), 178–87.

Lawlor, D. A., et al. (2005). "Avoiding Milk May Lower Diabetes Risk." *Diabetic Medicine* 22, 808–11.

Lee, I. et al. (1993). "Body Weight and Mortality: A 27-Year Follow-Up of Middle-Aged Men." *Journal of the American Medical Association* 270, 2823–28.

Levy, Thomas E. (2002). "Vitamin C, Infectious Diseases and Toxins." Xlibris Corporation.

Malkmus, George H. (2003). *God's Way to Ultimate Health.* Shelby, NC: Hallelujah Acres Publishing.

Malkmus, Rhonda. (1998). *Recipes for Life . . . from God's Garden.* Shelby, NC: Hallelujah Acres Publishing.

Manson, JoAnn E. (1987). "Body Weight and Longevity—A Reassessment." *Journal of the American Medical Association* 257, 353–58.

————. (2004, February 9). "The Escalating Pandemics of Obesity and Sedentary Lifestyle." *Archives of Internal Medicine,* 249–258.

Martinette, T. (2005). "Dietary Fiber and Blood Pressure." *Archives of Internal Medicine* 165, 150–56.

Martinez, Juan M. (2004, August/September). "The Euglycaemic Status and Infections: A Step to Real Immunity." *Townsend Letter for Doctors and Patients,* 90–97.

McBarron, Jan. (2000, July/August). "Is Fat Making You Unhappy?" *Essential Vitality,* 20–21.

McCollum, Elmer Verner. (1957). *A History of Nutrition: The Sequence of Ideas in Nutritional Investigation.* Boston: Houghton Mifflin.

Meyerowitz, Steve. (2002). *Water: The Ultimate Cure.* Summertown, TN: Book Publishing Company.

———. (2002, sixth edition). *Juice Fasting and Detoxification.* Summertown, TN: Book Publishing Company.

MIT Tech Talk. (2004, June 9). "The Skinny on Fat: MIT Researchers Establish First Link Between Eating and Aging."

Mokdad, A. H., et al. (1999). "The Spread of the Obesity Epidemic in the United States, 1991–1998." *Journal of the American Medical Association* 282(16), 1519–22.

Nedley, Neil. (1999). *Proof Positive.* Ardmore, OK: Nedley Publishing.

Nison, Paul. (2002). *Raw Knowledge.* New York: 343 Publishing Company.

———. (2002). *The Raw Life.* New York: 343 Publishing Company.

Null, Gary, et al. (2004, March). "Death by Medicine." Life Extension.

Olney, J. W. (1969). "Brain Lesions, Obesity and Other Disturbances in Mice Treated with Monosodium Glutamate." *Science* 165, 719–21.

Osteen, Joel. (2004). *Your Best Life Now.* New York: Warner Faith, Time Warner.

Oski, Frank. (1983). *Don't Drink Your Milk.* Brushton, NY: TEACH Services.

Ottoboni, Alice, and Fred Ottoboni. (2004, Winter). "The Food Guide Pyramid: Will the Defects Be Corrected?" *Journal of American Physicians and Surgeons,* 109–13.

Patenaude, Frederic. (2001). *Sunfood Cuisine.* San Diego: Genesis 129 Publishing.

Rippe, James M., and Susan Z. Yanovski. (1998, October 15). "Obesity—A Chronic Disease." *Patient Care,* 29–61.

Rogers, Sherry A. (2002). *Detoxify or Die.* Sarasota, FL: Sand Key Company.

Ross, Julia. (1999). *The Diet Cure.* New York: Penguin Books.

Ruser, Christopher B., et al. (2005, January). "Whittling Away at Obesity and Overweight." *Post Graduate Medicine,* 31–40.

Sandler, Benjamin P. (1951). *Diet Prevents Polio.* Milwaukee: The Lee Foundation for Nutritional Research.

Schwarzbein, Diana. (1999). *The Schwarzbein Principle.* Deerfield Beach, FL: Health Communications.

Sears, Barry. (1995). *The Zone.* New York: HarperCollins.

Shade, E. D., et al. (2004, June). "Frequent Intentional Weight Loss is Associated with Lower Natural Killer Cell Cytotoxicity in Postmenopausal Women: Possible Long-term Immune Effects." *Journal of the American Dietetic Association* 104(6), 903–912.

Shell, Ellen R. (2002). *The Hungry Gene.* New York: Atlantic Monthly Press.

Sheppard, K. (1993). *Food Addiction.* Deerfield Beach, FL: Health Communications.

Shikora, Scott A., and Edward Saltzman. (1998, November). "Revisiting Obesity: Current Treatment Strategies." *Hospital Medicine,* 41–49.

Siegel, Bernie S. (1986). *Love, Medicine and Miracles.* New York: Harper and Row.

———. (1989). *Peace, Love and Healing.* New York: Harper and Row.

Stitt, Paul A. (1981, 2nd edition). *Fighting the Food Giants.* Manitowoc, WI: Natural Press.

Street, B. (1992, January-February). "Carbohydrate Craving and Addiction." *The Counselor,* 12–14.

Taylor, Eric M., et al. (2005, January 26). "Obesity, Weight Gain, and the Risk of Kidney Stones." *Journal of the American Medical Association,* 455–62.

Thomas, D. (2001). "Mineral Depletion in Foods Over the Period 1940 to 1991." *The Nutrition Practitioner* 2(1), 27–29.

Valdes, A. M., et al. (2005 August). "Obesity, Cigarette Smoking, and Telomere Length in Women." *Lancet,* 366(9486), 662–4.

Visscher, Tommy L. S., et al. (2004, July 12). "Obesity and Unhealthy Life-Years in Adult Finns." *Archives of Internal Medicine,* 1413–20.

Weindruch, R. H., and R. L. Walford. (1988). *The Retardation of Aging and Disease by Dietary Restriction.* New York: Charles C. Thomas.

Weiss, Daniel. (2000, October). "How to Help Your Patients Lose Weight: Current Therapy for Obesity." *Cleveland Clinic Journal of Medicine,* 739–54.

White, James R. (1984). *Jump for Joy: The Rebounding Exercise.* New York: MacMillan.

Wolfe, David. (2002). *The Sunfood Diet Success System.* San Diego: Maul Brothers Publishing.

Wright, J. D., et al. (2004, February 2). "Trends of Intake of Energy and Macronutrients—United States, 1971–2000." *Morbidity and Mortality Weekly Report* 53, 80–82.

Yanovski, Jack A., and Susan Z. Yanovski. (1999, October 27). "Recent Advances in Basic Obesity Research." *Journal of the American Medical Association,* 1504–6.

———. (2003). "Calcium Modulation of Adiposity." *Obesity Research* 11, 375–76.

Zemel, Michael B. (1998, November). "Nutritional and Endocrine Modulation of Intracellular Calcium: Implications in Obesity, Insulin Resistance and Hypertension." *Molecular and Cellular Biochemistry,* 129–36.

Index

Page numbers followed by an *f* or *t* indicated figures or tables.

Buckwheat Milk, 293–94
Build Your Own Veggie Sandwich, 294–95
burdock, 122*t*
butter, 123*t*
butylenes glycol, 154
bypass, gastric, 222–26
Byrd, Randolph, 175

C

cabbage, 87, 93, 122*t*, 157
cabbage sprouts, 275
Caesar Salad, 302
Caesar Salad Dressing, 302–3
caffeine, 59, 64, 79–81, 265
Caffix, 264
calcium, 19, 44, 48, 62, 229–30, 242–43
calories, nutrient density and, 20
Campbell, T. Colin, 64, 74–75, 258, 273
Campbell, Thomas M., 258
cancer
    animal protein and, 73, 74–75
    barbecue and, 77
    body fat and, 33
    fiber and, 88
    Hunzas and, 18
    inflammation and, 128
    overweight and, 4, 13
    physical activity and, 188
    phytochemicals and, 86–87
    sugar and, 48
    toxins and, 149–50
    vitamin C and, 249
    vitamin D and, 252
cane sugar, 51
Canfield, Jack, 167, 183
canola oil, 69–70, 72, 123*t*, 270
canteloupe, 122*t*
carbamates, 141–42
carbohydrates, 104, 105–6, 132–33
carbon monoxide poisoning, vitamin C and, 249
carbonates, 242–43, 246
cardiovascular exercise, 189, 267, 272
carob, 70, 123*t*
carotenes, 197
carpets, 139, 151, 159
carrots, 87, 93, 123*t*
cars, 139, 159
casein. *See also specific diseases*
cashews, 122t
castile soap, 159
cauliflower, 87, 93, 122*t*, 157
CCNV, 165
celery, 93, 122*t*
cell function
causes of, 118–21
    essential fatty acids and, 126–27
    supplements and, 229–30, 230–32
    toxins and, 21
Cell Metabolism, 132
cellular medicine, introduction to, 7
celtic sea salt, 332

cereals, 67, 70, 139
cervical health, 22–23
Champion juicer, 330
chard, 123*t*
cheeses, 123*t*
chelates, 246
chemical sensitivity syndrome, overweight and, 4
chemicals, man-made. *See* toxins
chemistry, body, 11
cherimoya, 123*t*
cherries, 93, 122*t*
chestnut oil, 123*t*
chestnuts, 122*t*
chewing, 107–9
chick peas, 123*t*
chicken, 123t
children, 13, 29, 149, 276–78
China, 18–19, 74
The China Study, 64, 74–75, 258, 273
chips, 70
chives, 122*t*
chlorine, 149
chocolate, 70, 80, 198
cholesterol, 13, 113
chromium, sugar and, 44, 60, 62
chronic obstructive pulmonary disease (COPD), 203
chrysanthemum, 122*t*
chutney, 123*t*
cider vinegar, 122*t*
cilantro, 122*t*
cinnamon, 122*t*
Cinnamon Buckwheat Cereal, 312
circulation, physical activity and, 188
citrates, 243, 247
citrus, 122*t*
citrus squeezers, 330
clarified butter, 99–100, 122*t*
cleaning products, 154, 270, 273
climate, water and, 109–10
clover sprouts, 275
cocoa, 123*t*
coconut, 70, 123*t*
coconut oil, 99–100, 122*t*, 197, 270, 331
cod liver oil, 122*t*, 253
coenzyme Q10, 130, 157, 232, 243
coffee, 122*t*, 123*t*, 198, 264. *See also* caffeine
coffee creamer, 70
coffee grinders, 329
cohosh, 122*t*
Colbert, Don, 207, 275
cold-pressed oils, 70–71
colitis, 88
collard greens, 87, 122*t*
colon function, 88
color, food, 83, 85–87
Colorful Cabbage Delight, 306–7
coloring, food, 21
comfort foods, 40
computers, 159
concentration, sugar and, 45

organophosphates, 141–42
Oski, Frank, 78
Osteen, Joel, 164
osteoporosis, 18, 23–24, 74, 128, 149
overeating, 100–103
overweight
    causes of, 118–21 (*see also* Big Four, The)
    as a disease, 1–2, 5, 6–7, 9, 11–13, 21–25, 279
    fat burning and, 184–85
    genetics and, 136
    health status and, 13–15
    inflammation and, 128
    toxins and (*see* toxins)
oxides, 242–43, 246
oxygen. *See* breathing
oxygen bleach, 154

P

paint, 139
PAK. *See* pyridoxal alpha-ketoglutarate (PAK)
palm kernel oil, 123*t*
pans, cooking, 148
pantry items to have on hand, 331–32
papaya, 87, 93, 122t
parabens, 154
paradichlorobenzene, 152, 158–59
parchment paper, 330
Parkinson's disease, 150, 215
parsley, 122*t*
parsnips, 122*t*
partially hydrogenated oils, 69–70
particle-board, 159
pasta, 59, 67–68
pastries, 70
Patch Adams, 177
Patenaude, Frederic, 284
Pauling, Linus, 231
PCBs, 21, 94, 142, 158–59, 216
Peace, Love and Healing, 165
peaches, 93, 122*t*
peanut butter, 70
peanut oil, 72, 270
peanuts, 123t
pears, 93, 122t
peas, 123*t*
pecans, 123t, 331
peeling foods, 87
pellagra, 234
pepper, 122*t*
Perfect Body, 100–101
perfume, 139
permanent-press clothing, 159
Pero, 264
persimmon, 122*t*
persimmon juice, 123*t*
personal care products, 139, 140, 152–54, 270, 273
pesticides. *See also* toxins
    animal protein and, 76, 93
    hormones and, 216

organic food in response to (*see* organics)
overweight and, 21
as toxins, 141–42, 155
vitamin C and, 249
petrochemicals, supplements and, 241
pH, 121–25, 122t, 123t, 134, 244. *See also* acidity
Phase One menu plans, 286–88
Phase Three menu plans, 291
Phase Two menu plans, 288–90
pheasant, 123*t*
phenols, 154
phobias, sugar and, 45
phosphates, 246
phthalates, 21, 142, 154, 216
physical activity
    aging and, 186–87
    amount of, 272
    beginning, 262
    benefits of, 187–88
    eating and, 101
    fat burning and, 183–85
    importance of, 181
    modern society and, 17
    as pathway to NBFA Lifestyle, 28
    routine and, 189–90, 193
    Step One of the NBFA Lifestyle and, 265, 266
    Step Two of the NBFA Lifestyle and, 267
    Step Four of the NBFA Lifestyle and, 271
    Step Five of the NBFA Lifestyle and, 272
    tips for success, 192–94
phytochemicals, 84, 85–87, 95
pickled fruit, 123*t*
picolinates, 247
pine nuts, 123*t*
pineapple, 93, 122t
pineapple juice, 122*t*
pinto beans, 123*t*
Pirsig, Robert M., 183
pistachios, 123*t*, 331
pizza, 70, 79, 144–45
placebo effect, 164, 165–66
plantains, 93
plastics, 147
plums, 87, 93, 123*t*
plywood, 159
pollution, 201–4
polychlorinated biphenyls (PCBs), 21, 94, 142, 158–59, 216
poppy seeds, 122*t*
pork, 93, 123*t*
portion size, 117–18
potassium, 62, 80
potassium bromate, 154
potatoes, 93, 122*t*
pots, cooking, 148
poultry, pesticides and, 93
The Power of Focus, 167, 183
prayer, 163, 175–76
pregnancy, caffeine and, 80
preparation, NBFA Lifestyle and, 260–61

shampoo, 139, 140, 154, 158–59
shaving foams, 154
sheep cheese, 123t
shell fish, 123t
Shelton, Herbert, 275
shortening, vegetable, 69–70
Siegel, Bernie, 165, 166
sinus problems, mercury toxicity and, 23–24
skin disorders, 113, 191
sleep, 13, 23–24, 130, 132, 181, 198–99
slippery elm, 122t
snake bite, vitamin C and, 249
snow peas, 123t
soaps, 139, 158–59
soda
    acidity and, 123t, 124
    caffeine and (see caffeine)
    caloric content of, 42
    diet, 146
    with meals, 108
    Standard American Diet and, 17–18
    table salt as, 123t
sodium
    results of excess, 111, 118–21
    retention of, 48
    sea salt and, 122t, 332
    Standard American Diet and, 17
    sugar cravings and, 58
sodium cetyl sulfate, 154
sodium laureth sulfate, 154
sodium lauryl sulfate, 154, 158–59
soft drinks. See soda
soils, depletion of, 231
soluble fiber, 88
solvents, 21, 237
soups, 70
soy sauce, 122t
soybean oil, 69–70, 72, 252, 270
soybeans, 123t
Soymage Parmesan, 332
spaghetti sauce, 332
spaghetti squash, 68
spelt, 65, 67, 123t
spelt berries, 330
spices, 122t
Spicy Raw Nuts, 321
spider bite, vitamin C and, 249
spinach, 87, 93, 123t
spirituality, 175
Splenda, 61–62. See also artificial sweeteners
split peas, 123t
spray bottles, 329
sprouted-grain products, 66
The Sprouting Book, 275
sprouts, 76, 122t, 274, 275–76
squash, 68, 122t
squid, 123t
Standard American Diet, 16–18, 43–44, 74, 119, 127–28
starches. See carbohydrates
steaming baskets, 330

Step One of the NBFA Lifestyle, 263–66
Step Two of the NBFA Lifestyle, 267–68
Step Three of the NBFA Lifestyle, 268–70
Step Four of the NBFA Lifestyle, 270–72
Step Five of the NBFA Lifestyle, 272–74
Step Six of the NBFA Lifestyle, 274–76
steroids, 142
stevia, 52–53, 123t, 263, 265–66, 332
stimulants, 198
Stitt, Paul, 67
stoves, 152
strainers, 330
strawberries, 87, 93, 122t
stress, 30, 129–30, 181, 199–201, 268
stretching. See flexibility
string beans, 123t
sucanat, 122t
succinates, 247
sucralose, 61–62. See also artificial sweeteners
sucrose, 50
sugar
    acid-forming nature of, 44–45
    acidity and, 123t, 124
    artificial sweeteners and (see artificial sweeteners)
    genetics and, 216
    hidden sources of, 50–53
    hormones and, 49
    immunity and, 45
    impact on health and, 39–40, 43–44
    insulin and, 46–49
    mental health and, 45–46
    natural sugars and, 54–55
    as part of The Big Four, 41–42
    reducing the use of, 56–58
    soluble fiber and, 88
    Standard American Diet and, 17
    Step One of the NBFA Lifestyle and, 264
    substitutes for, 53–54
    white flour as, 64–66
    withdrawal from, 55–56
sugar and, elimination of, 58–60
Sugar Blues, 46
sugar cane syrup, 51
suicidality, serotonin and, 132
sulfates, 246
sulfite, 122t
sunflower oil, 69–70, 123t, 270
Sunflower Seed Milk, 293–94
sunflower seeds, 331
Sunfood Cuisine, 284
The Sunfood Diet Success System, 197
sunlight, Step Two of the NBFA Lifestyle and, 267
sunscreen, 154, 194–97
sunshine, 181, 194–97, 252–53
Sunshine Burgers, 332
Super Size Me, 81
supplements. See also specific vitamins/minerals
    cell function and, 230–32
    detoxification and, 157–58

About Health-e-America Foundation (HeAF) and TPED

Health-e-America Foundation (HeAF) is an educational nonprofit organization. Its mission is to use education to arrest and reverse our epidemic of chronic disease. HeAF is the sponsor of The Project to End Disease (TPED). There are TPED chapters in cities and towns across America. By attending regular TPED meetings, you can learn more about how to get well, stay well, and never be sick or fat again. If there is not a TPED chapter in your community, you can start one and help to put a stop to this tragic epidemic of chronic disease.

For more information on HeAF go to www.healthe america.org, or call 415-459-3686. To support this important work, tax-deductible donations can be sent to:

Health-e-America Foundation
P.O. Box 150578
San Rafael, CA 94915

Never doubt the power of small groups to change the world; indeed, it is the only thing that ever has.

—Margaret Mead, Anthropologist (1901–1978)

About the Authors

Raymond Francis, D.Sc., M.Sc., R.N.C., is a chemist, a graduate of MIT, an internationally recognized leader in the field of optimal health maintenance and the author of *Never Be Sick Again.* He is chairman and CEO of Beyond Health Corporation, a supplier of highly advanced health education and health-supporting products. He is also president of Health-e-America Foundation, national chairman of the Project to End Disease, publisher of *Beyond Health News,* and host and producer of the *Beyond Health* radio talk show. He lives in San Rafael, California. Contact him at: mail@beyond health.com.

Michelle King is a health writer, an editorial assistant for *Hippocrates* magazine, and the assistant to the director of Hippocrates Health Institute in West Palm Beach, Florida. She works with people to enhance their health by changing their diet and lifestyle, giving particular attention to those with weight-loss issues.